MW00529364

GAME PLAN

GAME PLAN

A Proven Approach to Work, Live, and Play at the Highest Level Possible—for as Long as Possible

Mike Mancias

WITH MYATT MURPHY

wm

WILLIAM MORROW

An Imprint of HarperCollins*Publishers*

This book is written as a source of information only. The information contained in this book should by no means be considered a substitute for the advice of a qualified medical professional, who should always be consulted before beginning any new diet, exercise, or other health program. All efforts have been made to ensure the accuracy of the information contained in this book as of the date published. The author and the publisher expressly disclaim responsibility for any adverse effects arising from the use or application of the information contained herein.

The material on linked sites referenced in this book is the author's own. HarperCollins disclaims all liability that may result from the use of the material contained at those sites. All such material is supplemental and not part of the book. The author reserves the right to close the website in his/her sole discretion following the end of 2024.

HarperCollins books may be purchased for educational, business, or sales promotional use. For information, please email the Special Markets Department at SPsales@harpercollins.com.

FIRST EDITION

Designed by Kyle O'Brien

Library of Congress Cataloging-in-Publication Data has been applied for.

ISBN 978-0-06-331643-0

24 25 26 27 28 LBC 5 4 3 2 1

Contents

GAME PLAN

Foreword

LeBron James

I first met Mike when I was just eighteen, right after I was drafted into the league and he was a summer league intern for the Cavaliers. I didn't see him again until my second year in the NBA, when the Cavs hired him as an assistant trainer. Back then, what immediately stood out was his demeanor and how punctual he was. Every single day, he came in hungry, super excited, and ready to work—just like I did. More importantly, he understood the value of longevity.

Staying in the game for as long as possible has always been a part of my mindset since middle school. I remember when I was thirteen, a friend of mine told me to play hard and have fun, but never forget to stretch.

Every.

Single.

Game.

I would stretch two or three times a day, not just before games but as soon as I'd wake up and right before bed. So that no matter how ready I was to play *that* day, I'd be just as ready to play tomorrow, the next day, and every day after that. Because I've always been one of those guys who realized that no matter how much talent you might have, when it comes to your skills, they can only get you so far. That if you wanted to have a long and sustainable career—that if you wanted to become legendary—you have to be available for your team. To do that, you always got to put the work in. No matter what—no excuses.

I heard about how Mike had interned with world-renowned performance coach Tim Grover and assisted with helping Michael Jordan during his comeback. He wasn't assigned to me when training camp started that

October, but when I saw him warming up some of the veterans on the team, I asked him, "Hey! Can I get some of that?"

As Mike tells it, that day he made the higher-ups nervous working with me when he was just the "new guy." But I saw something in Mike early on and we hit it off right from the beginning. We weren't just two young guys coming up the ranks in the NBA. We were two guys with goals, principles, and work ethics in perfect sync. And I needed someone who could not only challenge me but wasn't afraid to. Someone I could be comfortable with who always put in the work when it came to my health, training, and recovery. Every single day, no matter what—no excuses.

I've always felt like Mike was the guy for me because he believed just like I did that longevity starts by being consistent both on and off the floor. It's about centering yourself even when your head's not in the game, showing up prepared, and tackling each moment at the highest level possible. It's knowing the right way to learn from failure, because whether you like it or not—you will fail. And two decades later, we're still getting better together by learning on the fly, trusting each other to try new things that might work, and if they don't, then we just move on to something else. But most importantly, we ask ourselves what we can learn from this defeat. So when we cross that threshold again, we approach things differently and stand the best chance of being successful.

Even when I'm done playing the sport of basketball, I still plan on keeping my body as functional as possible by doing the right things. I'm staying in the game for as long as possible by being consistent with my training, my recovery, and eating as clean as I can—and a big part of that is because of Mike.

We live in a world where everyone's trying to figure out how they can become a better version of themselves, both physically and spiritually. But it doesn't matter whether you're an athlete or an inspiring one—or a mom, dad, brother, or sister just looking to be your best self. The movements, training, and experience Mike brings to the table truly benefit anyone because it's not just about athlete empowerment—it's about human empowerment.

I trust him with my career.

I trust him with my friendship.

I trust him with my body.

What we've learned together is a part of my DNA now—and it's not going anywhere.

—LeBron James

Introduction

What do you need to get from your body today?

How about tomorrow?

Or the next day, week, month, or year after that?

Do you need your body to be leaner? Stronger? More flexible and injury-proof? To be in the best shape it can possibly be today, tomorrow, and beyond so that you can enjoy a long and healthy life?

When you're a client of mine, these are questions you better be ready to hear on a regular basis.

I met LeBron James his second year in the NBA during the '04–'05 season, when he was looking for help with his training. It was easy to see that he was a very gifted and special athlete. Back then, he was able to achieve success through raw strength and traditional training and weight-lifting techniques. His training wasn't aimed at moving more efficiently or incorporating any preventative measures to avoid injury. There was no structure—no stretching regimen or nutritional plan, no pre- or post-game or half-time routine in place—beyond him just lacing up his shoes, hitting the court, and going two hundred miles an hour. I could see he was a blank canvas with literally every paint color available—it just wasn't organized the right way yet.

Our initial talk became the first of thousands we've had since, and over the last two decades, as his athletic trainer and recovery specialist, I've worked with him one-on-one nearly every single day of his career to keep him playing at his highest possible level. But on that first day with LeBron, I asked him that same question: *What do you need to get from your body today?*

His answer has evolved over the years. At first, he was simply looking for a better way to train and recover. Then he wanted to be the best in the league. Then the best ever. Then to stay the GOAT for as long as possible. And now he wants to remain healthy enough to play in the NBA with his son.

When you reflect on that question—not just each day, but before, during, and after certain crucial decision-making moments regarding your diet, activity, and recovery throughout your day—all the pieces needed to make your answer become a reality finally begin to fall into place. That's what moves you down the path of becoming more accountable, consistent, and successful.

Truth is, there is no "secret sauce" or "magic bullet" when it comes to health and wellness. We already know the essentials that enable the human body to be at its absolute best for as long as possible: Eat healthier, exercise more, and get enough rest. What separates the best from the rest is **figuring out the smartest way to remain consistent with what's been proven to work** so that you're less likely to quit or veer off course. **Because growth never ends and recovery never stops—unless you decide they do.**

LeBron was drafted into the NBA in 2003, along with fifty-seven other guys. Almost half of them didn't make it five years in the league. After fifteen years, six of them remained. As of this writing, LeBron is finishing his twenty-first season, and he's the only one left. Not only is he still playing, he remains one of the very best in the league. But if you think you can't reap the same resilience, think again. What my clients have needed physically, nutritionally, and mentally to maximize their abilities and prolong their longevity may have morphed over the years, but how I have them address certain choices in their lives hasn't. And now it's your turn to tackle the crucial decisions that affect your own life in the same way.

Look, most of us are not going to become professional athletes, but just because you're not paid to play a sport doesn't mean you're not expected to perform. People talk about LeBron's longevity—but let's talk about *your* longevity. What pushes *you* to stay in the game when others quit. Why do *you* need to be at your best right now and every day after that for as long as possible.

This program is the written culmination of two decades working with some of the world's top athletes and performers to maximize their potential, including LeBron James, two-time NFL All-Pro Myles Garrett, and award-winning superstar Usher. It's a program that covers all the bases regarding both functional movement and functional strength, allowing you to quickly and easily make your body stronger, more pliable, and injury-resistant to extend your longevity. This system incorporates the same tactics I use with all my clients, which allows anyone—athlete or otherwise—to work, live, and play at a higher level than they ever thought possible, for as long as possible. The comprehensive four-step method combines the smartest applications in mobility training, performance nutrition, and active recovery, holding you accountable at certain critical moments of each day so that you finally make the best choices for your health and wellness without fail—and live the best life possible. It's a plan that teaches you how to execute every decision regarding your longevity in four importantly crucial ways: You'll THINK each decision forward, you'll FOLLOW each decision through, you'll BREAK down what you did afterward, and finally, you'll REBUILD it better. This proven approach will change your attitude about failure so you'll understand and embrace that every loss is an opportunity to win.

So, what do you need to get from your body today?

Only you know the answer to that question, but I know how you can get it. So—let's do this.

CHAPTER 1

Mind First–Grind Later

If you're reading this, then you most likely have a history of trying to change your body for the better. So what happened? Why is it a history of "trying" instead of "succeeding"? I know why. It starts up top, because even though a client may seek me out to improve their body, we always begin with their brain.

I've met people who fail because they never invest in the right mindset before working toward their goals. They fail because they try to go it alone instead of bringing as many people to the table as possible. They fail because they never have a conversation with themselves beforehand about why they are taking this journey in the first place.

In order for my methods to work for you, there's something you need to do each and every morning. It's quick, I promise. The moment you wake up—not after breakfast or a few hours later, but the very second you open your eyes—ask yourself four questions:

1. Do I know what I want from my body today?
2. Is there a team ready to support me?
3. Am I prepared to lose?
4. Do I deserve success?

I'm going to get honest with you right now. If asking these questions feels silly, that already tells me which direction you're going—and it's a path that leads nowhere.

You see, a big part of how I get my clients to evolve is through evaluation. I ask my clients a lot of questions because it's the only true way to get right to the heart of why certain things are moving them forward and others are pulling them backward. It's those questions that help the client and I figure out together why they're not sticking with what they obviously know they should, as well as determine how to make a stronger connection with the things they're doing right so those things happen more frequently.

But I can't be there with you.

Instead, I'm counting on you to be there for yourself, which will require you to ask a lot of questions of yourself at different points throughout the day. That's a big part of how my program works. So if you have any problems with that, or have a hard time being honest with yourself, stop reading right now and come back to me when you're ready.

BACK SO SOON? GLAD YOU could join me—I mean that. Now, let's get serious.

Why are those four questions so important to me—and why are they so critical for you? Because it's how you answer that tells me—and tells you—if you're going to win or lose the day. If you can honestly say yes to all four, you're a winner before you've even begun. But say no to any of these questions—even just one of them—and I can pretty much guarantee that your chances of succeeding are a lot lower.

Here's why each question is so important:

Do I Know What I Want from My Body Today?

Is the answer no? If so, I can say with 100 percent certainty that it's not that you don't have expectations of your body—it's probably because you don't know where to begin. Instead of letting yourself become overwhelmed with all the things you're about to put your body through today, hone in on the most important thing. I call this your "bull's-eye." What is your bull's-eye for the day?

For LeBron, his bull's-eye might be a game or practice where he wants to play his best, or an event or function where he needs to present himself with confidence. For you, it may be to push yourself further in your workout, look unshakable in that board meeting, finish all that yard work that's long overdue, feel less achy and stiff than you usually do, play the back nine as strong as the front nine, or simply have enough energy to play with your kids after work. It's in there—that moment of your day when you need your body to be at its best above all other moments.

So what is your bull's-eye? What do you specifically need from your body that should be your center of attention for the day?

Is the answer yes? That's good, but you're not done yet. Even if you know which moment of the day you need your body to be at its best, I want you to take a step further and tell me *why* hitting that bull's-eye dead-center is so important. You can think of these reasons as the rings around your bull's-eye, keeping you focused on the target.

For example, if your bull's-eye is to be healthier and fitter, that's a start, but the real question is: Why do you want that in the first place? Is it because you want to look better in your clothes? Fine, that's one ring. Keep going. I want you to surround that bull's-eye with every single reason or benefit you can think of that's tied to that bull's-eye. If being healthier and fitter is your goal today, then a few more perks might include the following:

- It will allow you to do more things with your kids, friends, or other loved ones. (If so, then every single person you're thinking about is a ring.)
- It will help you feel more confident at work.
- It will lower some numbers that your doctor is concerned about. (If that's the case, then each health issue is its own separate ring.)
- It will improve your sex life.

I don't know what your rings are—only you do—but I want you to think of at least six separate reasons or benefits to surround your bull's-eye. If you feel like it, take it a step further by writing down your reasons on a piece of paper that you can carry in your pocket or tape up somewhere if you need a constant reminder throughout the day. But understand this: Don't expect that today's bull's-eye will be tomorrow's bull's-eye. It could change from month to month or even from day to day depending on what you have going on.

Your bull's-eye doesn't even have to always be tied to your health, wellness, or longevity. If you have a pick-up game after work and your bull's-eye that day is to play your best, that's perfect. I still want you to think about all the reasons why that matters to you on that day and surround it with as many rings as you can. Look, they can be selfish or selfless—I won't judge—but you're more likely to hit that bull's-eye if you remind yourself why you're aiming for it. Maybe the reasons are:

- You don't want to let down your teammates.
- You want your kids to see you play well.
- You won't be able to hit the gym, and this game is your exercise for the night.
- You just really want to beat the team you're playing against because they're cocky.

Seriously, no reason is considered a reach or ridiculous in my book, so long as it genuinely motivates you and lights a fire under your ass to get the job done. Because the more you can figure out what's honestly driving you toward that bull's-eye today, the more often you'll remind yourself throughout the day why that goal is so important. The more rings you can wrap around that bull's-eye, the more likely you'll be to fly straight and stay on target.

Is There a Team Ready to Support Me?

Is the answer no? Do I personally believe you have the strength to do this program without needing to rely on anyone but yourself? Of course, but any goal becomes much easier to achieve when others support you every step of the way.

Very few athletes go at it alone. Even in sports such as tennis, powerlifting, distance running, and so on, athletes may fly solo when it's time to compete, but behind the scenes, they still count on the encouragement and strength of coaches, trainers, mentors, and family. It's that team of individuals that helps create a backbone of consistency. When you have a support network, not only do you have a safety net of individuals ready to catch you when you fall, but you have a set of people you can rely on to hold you accountable. The more support you can surround yourself with *before* you start this journey—and have behind you every day—the easier it becomes to hit that bull's-eye because you're bringing others along for the ride.

So if you answered no, what I need you to do is start collecting rocks and dropping anchors. What do I mean by that? Look around at the people in your life—your colleagues, your friends, your relatives, and so on—and ask yourself how you would classify each of them.

- A **rock** is somebody who's optimistic and encourages you, gives you strength when you need it most, and genuinely listens to what you have to say (instead of talking over you). A rock has your back in moments when others don't, sees good things in you that sometimes you don't see in yourself, and always has your best interests at heart.
- An **anchor** is someone who's pessimistic and always complaining. They tend to reorient the conversation back to themselves, and they may silently compete against you. An anchor will make themselves scarce when you need them. These are the ones you need to avoid as often as possible and/or minimize how much time you're forced to spend around them. Obviously, there might be certain people who are much harder to avoid than others—a boss, a relative, or a neighbor, for example—but sometimes all it takes is looking at your day and thinking of ways that make it less likely to encounter them.

So what about those who fall in the middle? The neutral ones who aren't out there cheering you on but definitely not looking to tear you down either? Well, that's where the majority of people in our lives typically fall, which is entirely fine. So long as those individuals aren't negatively affecting you or making you feel self-conscious to implement my methods, they're harmless. In fact, count them up because it sometimes helps prove the point about how rare "true rocks" really are among everyone else who's around you every day.

Look, no matter what you tell yourself, you are, for the most part, in control of who you surround yourself with. Sure, certain negative co-workers or family members may be hard to escape at certain times, but typically, we decide who we orbit and, to a major degree, who gets to orbit us. You need to seek out and enlist as many people as possible who want you to succeed, who you can count on to help you go further because they have no agenda other than to see you triumph.

Is the answer yes? If you already have your rocks, then you need to tell every single one of them your intentions. Don't keep things to yourself, only relying on them at low points—make them an active part of the process. The more aware your rocks are about what you're about to embark on, the more likely you'll stick with it. So, with each rock:

Give them the scoop on exactly what you're doing. I don't want you to be vague but, rather, incredibly specific. In other words, don't just say you're trying my four-pronged approach toward diet, movement, and recovery. Tell them exactly how it works and how each day you're going to have a specific bull's-eye in mind. It's pretty hard not to stay on point when every day certain people might ask you, "Hey, what do you need to get from your body today?"

Grant them permission to call you out. This can be hard for some people, but if these are genuinely people you trust (people you know want you to flourish), give them free rein to point out when you might be aiming in the opposite direction of your bull's-eye.

Go out with (or be around) them as often as possible. Having a team of rocks that you never see makes it harder for them to hold you accountable, but it's not just that. If you're surrounding yourself with those who truly care about you, seeing them often reminds you of why you're doing this in the first place—to be your best self not just for you, but for others as well.

Get them on board if you can. Look, misery may love company, but nothing beats accomplishing something alongside someone else. The more people you can pull on board to follow my approach, the more the process becomes a team effort, turning your rocks into like-minded strivers like yourself.

Am I Prepared to Lose?

A lot of life is nothing more than a series of wins, losses, and draws. Sure, winning's great, and a draw can sometimes be hard to swallow or a blessing, depending on whether we expected to pull off a victory or a loss. But losing? Let's face facts—no one likes to lose. But it's all part of the game, and depending on how graceful and attentive you are when you deal with failure, you can decide whether you lose or win the next time.

Is the answer no? Then guess what—you've already lost. Because the most successful people in every walk of life have lost along the way and continue to lose each day.

It doesn't matter if it's work, relationships, family dynamics, exercise, health, or diet; we all experience moments in which we finish first and others where we come in last. Both hardships and tough times occur right alongside moments of celebration and victory because it's never one continuous journey upward or, fortunately, never one ongoing, out-of-control trek downward.

Basketball is a good metaphor for life. No team has ever existed (or will ever exist) that's won every game—and there's never been (and never will be) a player who's made every single shot they've taken. We readily accept that this is true; perfection is statistically impossible. Yet when it comes to ourselves, we often forget that it's statistically impossible for us not to fail. That pressure only leads to disappointment, preventing you from treating each failure and mistake for what they truly are—opportunities to learn so that you perform better the next time.

Is the answer yes? Then that's great because you will lose—in fact, get ready to lose a lot. What you clearly understand is that losing and failing are not the same thing. Each time you lose, it's a chance to address that loss and turn it into a crucial teaching moment. The only way you'll ever fail with this program is not taking the time to listen to what each mistake made is trying to tell you.

Do I Deserve Success?

I mean it—why you? I make this the fourth and final question with clients because this is that game-changer moment—the answer that makes or breaks your mindset.

Is the answer no? You're not alone. It doesn't happen often, but I have had a select few clients in the past surprise me with that very answer. It's not an easy thing to hear, just as I'm sure it's not an easy thing to say, but if there's any good to come from it, it's this: With that one answer, you've just figured out why you've probably always struggled with reaching your goals—wellness, longevity, whatever the case may be.

If you don't feel like you deserve something, I can almost guarantee that you won't get it, end of story. That's not rocket science—that's just reality. Because if you don't believe it's your turn to be next in line for success, then you've never gotten in line in the first place. If that's you, then you need to ask yourself why that is and address it by whatever means necessary (because whatever you need to do to see that you're worthy of success is beyond my realm of expertise), but then please come back to me.

However, before you do, let me say this: I've asked you to collect as many rocks as possible, but the most important rock you need to pick up first is yourself. You need to be your own rock. You need to be accountable to yourself, and with this book, you will learn to be.

Is the answer yes? Perfect, because I couldn't agree more. What you're hoping to achieve isn't a selfish goal. It's wanting to get more from your body for as long as possible so you can live a better life, both for yourself and for those you care about. Everybody deserves that—you deserve that—and now, you're about to have that.

So are you willing to work harder than those around you? Ready to trust the plan and not rush the process? Prepared to put in the time that it takes? Most important, are you excited about what you're about to do?

Good, because now you're in the right mindset—exactly where you need to be—so let me show you how we're going to achieve that success together.

CHAPTER 2

Think, Follow, Break, and Rebuild

LeBron and I always make sure we're the first ones at the gym. We're also the first to step into the arena, sometimes even before any of the stadium workers punch in. This not only sets the tone for the day, but it gives us plenty of time to plan and scrutinize everything we hope to accomplish. Because here's the truth: Things don't just come naturally to most super-high performers, in any field. They have to work for it. They know it's the details that determine who plods through life without making a mark and who excels.

Most people typically fail with their performance and longevity goals because it's not just about being able to say, "I did it!" It's about asking yourself certain questions before you even do whatever "it" might be and checking in with yourself to make sure you're doing "it" in the smartest way possible. But above all else, it's reminding yourself at every opportunity why you're even doing "it" in the first place.

High performers understand this, which is why those in the know break down their daily habits in a way that lets them quickly see what they can improve and what they should put an end to. They remind themselves "in the moment" of their successes so that they become more likely to repeat their wins and forgive themselves for (and learn from) their failures so they're less likely to repeat their losses.

Think, Follow, Break, and Rebuild

I need you to understand above all else that my method isn't about following a specific diet or tossing in a series of quick fixes. Instead, it's about leveraging certain clutch moments in your day to rethink and recalibrate your life. I especially like to focus on:

1. What you EAT
2. When you MOVE
3. How you MEND

I believe in honesty, and when you apply that to your life during these moments, your life literally has little choice but to improve. It takes not being afraid to look objectively and truthfully at everything you do and every decision you make regarding improving yourself. If you can't do that, then this book will not pull you out of the hole you're presently in. But if you're ready to be honest with yourself—to be honest with me—that honesty will become the heart of everything you're about to do with me, just as it is for my clients. Because when it comes to LeBron and the rest of my clients:

1. They THINK . . . it forward

What I do with those I work with is have them boil down their day and get them really thinking about certain choices they'll eventually have to make about their diet, exercise, and healing habits long before making them. For example, I won't ask just what they plan on having as a meal or snack, but precisely when and where they plan on eating that meal or snack. Instead of just reminding them they'll be exercising that day or which therapeutic tactics I need them to do, I'll make them contemplate things such as what could pull them off course or affect their performance. That pre-prep isn't just to ensure they have everything they may need at their disposal, but it's a mental walkthrough that reminds them what they're about to do and why they are doing it, so they approach each task with the best mindset.

2. They FOLLOW . . . it through

Knowing what you must do and actually *doing* it are two entirely different things. It's not that most of us don't know what healthy habits we should be practicing—it's that we're slow to incorporate those healthy habits into our lives and, most important, be consistent with them. I give my clients the game plan—blueprints that reveal the most intelligent activity choices, healthiest nutritional habits, and most effective recovery hacks that promote longevity—and expect them to execute it.

3. They BREAK . . . it down

After each meal is eaten, each workout is over, and each recovery tactic is completed, I don't let my clients rest on their laurels. That's when the real work begins. I have them openly acknowledge what went wrong and what went right. I make them assess without any guilt how they did, what got in the way, what they should be proud of, and how much they really brought to the table.

4. They REBUILD . . . it better

Finally, I have my clients use that self-reflection to reshape their next meal, their next workout, and their next opportunity to heal and recover. It's a strategy that enables them to instantaneously improve on what they just did so that they continuously see maximum results.

It's this constant renewal that makes my method possible to continue for weeks, months, years—the rest of your life—without it ever becoming boring. Every day is different because that's how life works. But with time, you'll learn to foresee possible failures before they happen, know how to adjust when certain failures are impossible to avoid, and be able to boost yourself back up if you do take a loss. Each day, you'll remind yourself of your strengths, play them to your advantage, and reward yourself the right way to improve your odds of crushing it the next day.

Eat, Move, and Mend

As I mentioned earlier, these three areas in life are the most important to continuously stay on top of in order to live up to your greatest human potential. That's why I've divided up the book into three parts—Eat, Move, and Mend—allowing you to quickly and easily apply the Think, Follow, Break, and Rebuild strategy to any situation throughout your day.

Now, do you have to do all three sections *exactly* as prescribed? I do, since all three work with and build on one another. However, if you follow a very specific (and healthy) nutritional plan that's similar—or if there are certain suggestions of mine you can't follow due to allergies, health concerns, or personal reasons—I encourage you to check with your doctor (or dietitian) and modify certain portions of my nutritional blueprint.

However, I encourage you to do the Move section exactly as I've suggested (once you have approval from your doctor to do so). This mobility and performance regimen is the very backbone of everything I do with LeBron and other clients, and no matter what exercise program you already follow or how active your lifestyle is, Move will work behind the scenes to enhance what you're presently doing.

Before you begin the program, here's one final piece of advice: Breaking down your daily habits the way I'm asking you to will be hard and time-consuming at first. The longer you stick with it, though, the easier it will get. Before you know it, you'll find that you won't need to focus on the details quite so diligently. Healthier habits will suddenly be second nature to you. You'll quickly become as accountable in these three crucial areas in the same way my high-performers are, a level that's not only attainable but deserved—because you are just as valued as they are.

Even though the events in your life—your personal bull's-eyes—might not be the playoffs or a concert in front of tens of thousands, they're just as important because they matter to you and because this is your life. The more skilled you are at instantly accessing and addressing your nutrition, activity, and recovery choices, the faster and more effectively you can enhance your performance and longevity with less stress and better results, allowing you to perform at your best and have a better life.

That's what I want for every client and that's what I want for you. If that's also what you want for yourself, then let's get started.

PART I

EAT

CHAPTER 3

Think It Forward

I already know what you're thinking: Mike, if the mobility and performance regimen is the backbone of this book, then why aren't you starting with the Move portion? The answer is this:

First, food supplies energy, and you need energy to exercise—period! If there's not enough fuel in your gas tank, your body will stay parked more than you'll be taking it on the road.

Additionally, putting the best fuel into your tank by making smarter nutritional choices will allow you to bring more energy and focus to the Move portion of my program so that you reap more results. I need your body to have all the nutritional materials it needs on a daily basis to both rebuild and repair muscle, as well as curb or quell any urges you may have to reach for unhealthy and/or excessive amounts of food.

Finally, these next four chapters may fall under the category of *eating*, but you'll be applying my four-step program toward what you *drink* as well. Maintaining ideal hydration is paramount to the plan (you'll understand the many reasons why shortly), which is something these earlier chapters will help you quickly master.

All that said, let's get into it!

AS YOU'RE READING THIS, YOU likely ate or drank something a few hours ago. You probably plan on eating or drinking something after putting this book down. You might literally be throwing something back as you're turning these pages. So tell me—why did you choose (or why will you choose) that meal or snack?

When you're striving for longevity and performance, being responsible in all areas of your life is crucial—including nutrition. Yet when most people reach for something to eat or drink, it's rarely with longevity in mind. Frequently, it's for the wrong reasons entirely, such as the following reasons:

We're ignoring what our body's really asking us for. Often, what we are craving to eat or drink can be a sign that we need to consume something else entirely. For example, sometimes when you feel hungry, you might actually be thirsty instead, since your body usually receives a certain percentage of its daily water intake from the foods you eat. Or you could be craving salty foods because your body is dehydrated and short of electrolytes, specifically sodium.

Other times, you might be overeating starchy, sweet, and high-fat foods because your body is desperately in need of shut-eye. Science has long proven that not getting enough adequate sleep disrupts the balance of ghrelin, the hormone that increases your appetite by telling your brain it needs energy, and leptin, the hormone that suppresses your appetite by telling your brain it has enough energy at its disposal.

We're satisfying something besides our stomachs. There are plenty of times we reach for food for reasons that have nothing to do with being hungry or what our bodies need. When was the last time you ate fried foods from a carnival or boardwalk simply because it triggered a specific memory from your past? Or drank way more than you had planned on, only because you didn't want to bail on a night out with your buddies? Or reached for a bag of potato chips and found you had eaten your way down to the bottom just because you were bored or stressed?

Emotions can play a huge part in why we eat a lot of the garbage we know is garbage. That type of impulse eating gets in the way of putting the right foods in you—foods that match the personal goals you have for yourself in terms of performance and longevity.

We're starving—for time. When we're in a rush, the nutritional choices we make are usually decided by whatever foods are easiest to reach for.

Unfortunately, what's most convenient is typically the least healthy for us—and that's what gets most people in serious trouble.

Even the most conscientious eaters can fall victim to the worst foods possible when highly processed snacks or meals are what's at the ready when the clock is ticking. To make matters worse, being pressed for time leaves most of us feeling stressed, which causes your body to process whatever you're eating less efficiently, since stress shuts down digestion. That means you're getting even fewer nutrients from whatever valueless foods you're consuming in a pinch.

We're worried about our *form*—and not *performance*. How many people do you know that starve themselves to look better on the beach or fit into that smaller size dress? It's all too common, but that deprivation comes at a price, particularly if you're not getting enough of the nutrients your body needs.

Here's the thing: Most athletes aren't as concerned about the aesthetics of their physiques. Their goal is for their body to perform at—not look—its best. Makes sense, right? And yet, many of the most impressive athletes have incredible physiques anyway. Starving yourself to have six-pack abs isn't going to help you make a three-point shot or catch a forty-yard pass.

When you eat with performance first and foremost in your mind—when you spend a few seconds questioning whether what's about to hit your stomach is helping or hurting you—an enviable body pretty much develops on its own without too much thought involved. But instead of just *looking* like you can take care of business, you're literally fueling your body so that it *can* take care of business.

What to Think Through . . .

Before Starting This Program

I have all my clients follow the same nutritional blueprint, one that allows them to pull off what they're best at with as much energy and focus as possible for as long as possible. If the word *blueprint* sounds intimidating or complicated, trust me when I say that what I'll be proposing in the next chapter is not torturous or overwhelming. It's about following a few simple rules and consistently making the best possible choices when it's time to fuel your body. But I will say a few things right off the bat:

This isn't a weight-loss diet. I'll say it again: This isn't a diet. I need you to burn that into your brain. The moment I start explaining the type of foods a client should eat for longevity and performance, they'll often ask, "So how many pounds will I lose?" That is not what this is about. This is strictly about eating for longevity and performance by reaching for nutrient-dense foods that supply your body with everything it needs to stay energized and rebuild itself. I can't promise you you'll lose weight, but what I can guarantee is that you will feel and move much better than before.

This isn't some thirty-, sixty-, or ninety-day routine. When we talk about changing how and what we eat, there's often a timeline attached to it. But this isn't some fad diet I'm expecting you to adhere to for a certain number of days—this is a framework that I encourage you to incorporate for life. Because what I'm going to share with you isn't tied into today's latest trend. It's built around how your body works and what it needs, and those mechanics and essentials have been in place for as long as mankind's been on Earth.

This isn't the end of what you eat now. This is a framework that's flexible. Am I going to ask you to immediately give up every taco Tuesday, after-dinner dessert, or beers with your buddies from now until you breathe your last breath? No. You're still going to have access to all the things you love to eat and drink. But I can promise you this—you will begin to rethink how often you reach for the foods that aren't that friendly to your longevity.

Are You Making It Easier—or Harder—to Eat Better?

In sports, it's all about the numbers. When you can leverage certain numbers to work in your favor, you win more often. Nutrition is the same way.

Change the stats on your refrigerator and pantry. Look inside your fridge and pantry and take a quick tally of everything in them. For each food you know is healthy, add a check in one column. If it's something you know is not, give it a check in another column. And if you're not sure for now if what you're holding in your hand is good or bad for you, give it a check in a third column. Now, add each column up separately, then add up all three numbers together. You should have four numbers to play with: the good (G), the bad (B), the unsure (U), and the total amount of everything in your refrigerator and pantry (T). Here comes the fun part, and if you're not great at math, grab a calculator:

1. **Divide G by T, then move the decimal point to the right two spaces.** The number you're left with is not only the percentage of healthy foods kept in your house, but also, in a way, the chances that you'll even eat something healthy in the first place. For example, let's say you found 47 healthy things among the 162 items in your refrigerator. 47 ÷ 162 = .2901. Move the decimal point over two spaces and you have 29.01 (or 29 percent).
2. **Divide B by T, then move the decimal point to the right two spaces.** The number you're left with is the percentage of unhealthy foods you're giving a home to, as well as the odds you'll reach for that nasty stuff the next time you head in the icebox.

What about the foods you're unsure of? We can ignore them for now, because the more familiar you become with what you're consuming, that number will naturally start to decrease. And is this an exact science? No, of course not, but it does quickly bring to light what you surround yourself with and have access to. And as you do this (ideally every one to two weeks right before you go food shopping), it also gives you numbers to compare and compete against.

Am I saying you need to clear out everything in your kitchen that's unhealthy? Please. That would be irresponsible and downright cruel of me to ask of you, because who doesn't like bad-for-you food on occasion? All I really want you to do is look at those ratios as they stand right now and challenge yourself to swing them a little bit more in a better direction.

You might ask why I'm not hitting you with a specific stat to shoot for, such as 50 or 60 percent or higher. I mean, in a perfect world, the ideal percentage would be 100 percent, right? But that's not a perfect world because it's both not possible (because it's too strict) and not productive (because it's no fun!).

The athletes I work with are at the top of their game and need to be always firing on all cylinders. But sometimes that comes at the aid of a less-than-healthy snack right before a big event. For example, I train some of the most chiseled, most powerfully strong individuals in pro football today—and it's not uncommon to see them sneak in a bag of candy to our workouts to reach for in between sets. This aids them in feeling good and puts them in the right frame of mind to perform. So those unhealthy snacks tucked away can come out to play once in a while.

It's normal to have bad foods floating around—hell, you don't want to see what's tucked away in my pantry—but what's important to me is getting you in the habit of reducing your instant access to unhealthy foods. Keeping an eye on that percentage every week will make you consistently aware of what could be tempting you to eat poorly more often.

Change the stats of your route. We've all gone out of our way for bad food. Maybe it was driving an extra ten miles to hit that certain hot dog joint or bagel spot where they give you a slab of cream cheese an inch thick. But for the most part, we tend to be creatures of habit, always traveling from point A to point B along the same path. Even if you travel often—and trust me, I know what that's like being on the road with LeBron—you probably take the same routes, see the same sights, and stop at the same places to eat in between.

If the route you usually take to get to wherever you need to go swings you past a greater percentage of unhealthy restaurants, convenience stores, fast food places, or any spot that's too hard to resist, then change the stats by modifying your route slightly so you're less likely to stop there when hunger hits. If that's not possible, explore ahead of time what other options exist along that route so you're less likely to buy something unhealthy on impulse.

What Do the Next Three Days Look Like for You?

With LeBron, I like to ask him what his week looks like so we can plan accordingly. But sh*t happens, as they say. The reality of life is that every few days something different is thrown at you that you didn't expect.

In terms of thinking forward about diet, the same rules apply. Some people love to plan out their entire week, but when was the last time you had the best intentions of eating healthy Monday through Friday—and then a jam-packed Wednesday completely sidetracked your plans? Point being, when you plan *too* far ahead with your diet, something inevitably gets in the way, and when that happens, it can leave you feeling like a failure or reaching for whatever's convenient in the moment. Convenient options, for the most part, are never the healthiest choice.

That's why I prefer having clients look three days down the road and no further than that. Eating what's best for longevity and performance is all about remaining accountable, and it's much easier to stay accountable for just a few days than for an entire week—or, like so many lifestyle programs, for an entire month. Thinking forward in smaller three-day bursts not only keeps the whole task from feeling like too much of a chore, but it causes far less frustration when you fail and fall off the wagon with food. And you will fail, because we all do.

Think of it this way: When you plan things out for an entire week, you might have six great days, screw up the seventh, and then feel so guilty for messing up that last day that you never give yourself credit for the six days you succeeded. But by thinking things through just a few days ahead, you'll feel those moments of success a lot more often (fewer days means less margin of error) and if/when you do blow your diet, you'll find it's not as big a deal to move on.

In the next chapter, I'm going to explain what to eat and how often, but once you have those details, it's important to make sure your diet remains as flexible as possible. The easier it is for you to adapt when life has other plans, the less often your nutrition will be sidetracked—and the more focused and on point you'll be with your personal goals.

So . . . what do the next three days look like for you?

Despite life having other plans for us sometimes, for the most part, if we take a few moments to think about it a few days ahead, we're given a heads-up about what could potentially sidetrack us. That's why every three days, I want you to grab your calendar to see if there are any events, dates, holidays, barbecues, or anything else that could sideline your efforts over the next seventy-two hours. Do you have a road trip coming up? Is there a business meeting that's probably going to last longer than it really needs to? Is your kid's soccer game going to interfere with your supper plans? Will there be an afternoon or evening when you'll be out and won't have access to healthier foods? You can prepare for any problems before they begin by anticipating your options three days ahead of time.

What to Think Through . . .

Before Every Meal or Snack

Everybody talks about eating healthy as a matter of having enough willpower and discipline. That might be true, but how much of either trait you have often depends on how smart you are about what you're seconds away from gobbling up. Instead of going through the motions and just eating what you're told to eat, you need to have a deeper connection with what's healthy for your body in particular and how it affects you in a positive way. With clients, I get them to make that connection by having them consider a few things before they consume anything.

How Do You Feel in *This* Moment?

You're reaching for food or something to drink for a reason, but what you need to get to the heart of is whether it's for the right reason. Before you decide on *what* you're going to eat—whether that's grabbing something out of the fridge, strapping on an apron and playing chef, buying something from a convenience store, or ordering off the menu in front of you—you need to figure out *why* you're eating in the first place. Be honest with yourself when it comes to the following four questions:

1. **Where would you rank your hunger?**
   (1 being not hungry at all; 10 being absolutely starving):
   1 2 3 4 5 6 7 8 9 10
2. **Where would you rank your thirst?**
   (1 being not thirsty at all; 10 being completely parched):
   1 2 3 4 5 6 7 8 9 10
3. **Where would you rank your energy level?**
   (1 being the least alert; 10 being the most alert):
   1 2 3 4 5 6 7 8 9 10
4. **Where would you rank your stress level?**
   (1 being completely chill; 10 being seriously distressed):
   1 2 3 4 5 6 7 8 9 10

Where would I like to see those numbers fall?

- **Hunger:** Ideally, you should be right in the middle (around a 5 or 6), since not being hungry would make me wonder why you're eating in the first place, while being extremely hungry typically causes most people to either make poorer nutritional choices and/or eat more than their body really needs.
- **Thirst:** The lower the better when it comes to this number. By the time you're thirsty, your body is already dehydrated and that's not a place I ever want you to be.

- **Energy:** This is one where there is no right answer. For example, your energy level might be extremely low, but it could be because it's the end of the day or that you overexerted yourself exercising or playing a sport—and not because you necessarily need to eat. I just want you to have this number in your head for later when you gauge your energy levels after you've eaten.
- **Stress:** Again, the lower the better, but I want you to track this because of just how powerful emotional eating can be. We often don't recognize when we are stress eating because, well, we're too busy thinking about whatever is stressing us out in the first place.

Do I want you writing these numbers down on a piece of paper or plugging them into your phone? Yes, unless you have a photographic memory, it will make it much easier later when you refer back to these numbers after you've eaten (I'll explain later the reasons why). More important, do I expect you to do this every time you eat or drink something? Again, the answer is yes. What takes no more than a few seconds can (and will) play a big part in helping you make smarter food choices both in the moment and down the road.

Is This Food Honestly Helping Me Function?

Every time you sit down for a meal, pull something out of the fridge, or grab anything to eat or drink from the time you wake up until you hit the bed, the answer to this question must be yes. You need to know that there is a return on investment with what you're about to consume.

Now, I know what you're thinking: How can I expect you to have the answers to some of these questions if you're not a nutritionist or dietitian? Am I expecting you to know every single nutrient in everything you're eating and drinking, as well as know exactly what each nutrient offers and how it affects you? Of course not. That sort of minutia can be mind-numbing, and trying to follow that strict of a path is the fastest way to get to a place where you no longer care about what you're eating. Besides, you don't have to have a degree to know what's good for you. It doesn't take a diploma in dietetics to differentiate the good from the bad. All I want you to do is feel confident that what you're about to eat or drink is beneficial to your body, even if you don't know all the details why.

So how do you do that? Ask yourself the following five questions beforehand:

1. Is this as "clean" as possible?
2. Is this helping my body repair itself?
3. Is this improving my health?
4. Is this the right amount of food?
5. Am I proud of what I'm about to consume?

Is this as "clean" as possible? I'm not talking about whether you've washed the apple you're about to eat (although, please, do wash your fruits and vegetables). I mean, is whatever you're eating or drinking as free as it can be of anything artificial (preservatives, sweeteners, chemicals, etc.) or unnecessary (sauce, breading, toppings, and so on). The fewer ingredients on the label, the better.

Is this helping my body repair itself? How would you know that? Just look at how many grams of protein it has. Protein—the macronutrient found in meat, fish, eggs, dairy, nuts, and seeds—is known for building and maintaining lean muscle, but it's also responsible for growing and repairing every single cell in your body. Your bones, tendons, ligaments, cartilage, meniscus, skin—you name it—all rely on protein. And unlike carbohydrates and fat, protein is the only macronutrient your body can't store. That's why it's vital that it be a part of every meal or snack, even if building big muscles isn't your goal.

Is this improving my health? This question will be easier to answer once you've read the next chapter and learned what should be present in every meal or snack. But it's also one I like to have clients consider before every meal because it forces them to continuously learn.

What do I mean by that? Think about it this way: If I asked you to prove why the last thing you just ate was healthy for you, what would you tell me? But more important—how do you know it's true? I've had clients swear that something was good for them because it said "No Added Sugar" on the package. They didn't realize that only meant "no sugar was added during processing"; the food still contained massive amounts of sugar!

Having you answer this question forces you to defend your "yes." I don't want you to assume anything is healthy—I expect you to prove it as if I'm standing right in front of you. The more practiced you become at this, the more educated you'll become about the foods that most often find their way onto your plate.

Is this the right amount of food? Again, I'll share with you the optimal ballpark amount in grams of protein, carbohydrates, fiber, and healthy fats in the next chapter, which will make answering this question a lot easier. But this is also a question just as easily answered with common sense. If you're getting glances (or, worse yet, praise) for filling up your plate beyond its means and/or going back for seconds or thirds, consider the fact that you're most likely taking in more than your body technically requires.

Am I proud of what I'm about to consume? Look, I'm not expecting you to beam with pride every time you take a bite, but if you're experiencing any ounce of shame or guilt about what's in front of you, then there's probably a reason for it. Granted, there are always exceptions to this rule—having a slice of birthday cake or not being able to say no to that heavy meal your grandmother slaved over—but we all know the difference between what we can say no to and what we may need to temporarily accept in the moment.

OKAY, ENOUGH PREP WORK! NOW that you know the details regarding what you need to be thinking about *before* you eat, it's time to learn about what to throw back. Hope you're hungry!

CHAPTER 4

Follow It Through

Early in my career, I worked under Tim Grover, Michael Jordan's trainer, and began to develop the method I preach today. From Tim, I learned Jordan's philosophy on food: *Eat like a bird—just enough to fly.*

It is a simple mantra that has stuck with me because it holds true. When you don't overthink the process of eating but instead remind yourself to eat just enough to fly, you find you can go farther and higher than you ever thought possible.

What does that mean in the context of *your* diet? It means eating light, fresh, and as clean as you can. It means taking in a smart mix of macronutrients so that you feel fuller while eating less, a nutritional arrangement that provides you with all-day energy and everything your body needs to build muscle and repair itself so you remain in a constant state of healing. It means eating in a way that allows you to perform at your best. When you consistently do that, you'll find that the amazing physique, the lower cholesterol, and the additional years on top of your game—well, they sort of come along for the ride.

If that sounds like a lot of work, well, it can be if you overthink it—but it doesn't have to be overwhelming. All I'm asking you to do is make sure that every meal or snack contains one serving of protein, one serving of complex carbs, and one serving of healthy fats, as well as water. To be more specific:

- **One serving of high-quality protein** (either through meats—poultry, beef, pork, or fish—dairy products, or a combination of grains and legumes).
- **One serving of complex carbohydrates** (from fruits and vegetables and/or certain types of grains, such as oats, brown rice, or quinoa).
- **One serving of healthy fats** (which might already come with your protein serving, or can be added in separately through other sources, such as nuts, seeds, or certain types of oils, like olive, canola, or sunflower oil).
- **A minimum of 8 to 12 ounces of water** (which I'll get into in a bit).

A big reason most people tend to eat more than their body needs (and pack on more body fat as a result) is because they aren't eating the right balance of proteins, carbohydrates, and fats. When you eat all three within the same meal or snack, it provides you with a steady stream of energy because protein, carbohydrates, and fats are each digested by your body at varying speeds.

Carbohydrates are digested and utilized at a much faster pace than protein, which is part of the reason you might still feel hungry after throwing back a carb-rich meal. Fat takes the longest to break down, which explains why so many of us tend to eat too much of a fatty food before finally feeling satisfied. Protein is the "in-between" when it comes to energy—it takes much longer for your body to digest protein compared to carbohydrates, but it's more readily broken down into energy when compared to fat.

Consuming all three together ensures that you'll always have enough of each macronutrient in your system, which in turn provides your body with a steady stream of energy that will leave you feeling fuller longer while eating less food. You're far less likely to experience the up-and-down energy levels that can trigger binge eating—or even worse, cause your body to release insulin, which can cause you to store some of those calories as unwanted body fat.

Now, am I expecting you to nail this combo every single time you sit and chow down? Not at all. Remember what I said—and expect me to say it a few more times before this book is done: You *will* fail sometimes and that's okay. So long as you do your best to stay consistent with this rule of thumb most of the time, you're well on your way toward your longevity goals.

Let me give you a little more motivation on why you shouldn't skip any of these four elements: protein, complex carbohydrates, healthy fats, and water.

Protein

I'm a huge believer in protein at every meal *and snack*. I stress *snack* because many times, the foods we typically grab between meals to keep ourselves satiated tend to be nothing but carbohydrates. But every time you do that, every time you leave protein on the bench, you're preventing your body from healing and rebuilding itself.

You see, you have about 37 trillion cells in your body, and protein—well, there's a little bit of protein in every single cell. It's the second most common molecule you have in your body (water takes first place), and even though most associate it with their muscles, and rightfully so—your muscles are made up of about 20 percent protein and 80 percent water—your body desperately needs protein to produce practically everything. Not only is it used to build and maintain lean muscle, but it's needed to accomplish the exact same tasks for your bones, blood, hair, nails, skin, organs, cartilage, meniscus, tendons, ligaments, and other tissues. The macronutrient also comes in other forms (including antibodies, enzymes, hormones, and other important chemicals that assist with growth, function, and development) and assists your body in regulating the flow of water between blood vessels and surrounding tissues, fighting off disease-carrying bacteria and viruses, and, directly or indirectly, carrying out nearly every chemical reaction within your cells.

With all that responsibility on protein's shoulders, you would think I'd want you to eat as much as humanly possible, but there's a catch: Your body can process only 25 to 40 grams each meal. Once it has what it needs, it breaks any extra protein down and stores it as body fat. To make matters worse, that conversion process forces your liver and kidneys to work harder than necessary. Whenever your body breaks down protein, it has to remove nitrogen from the molecule, as well as any leftover ammonia that's a byproduct of the process. Both of those actions put stress on these two organs, so to keep them from working more than they should, being smart about eating just the right amount of protein is best.

Carbohydrates

Just like protein is thought by many to be a one-dimensional macronutrient capable of only one thing, carbohydrates suffer from a similar misunderstanding. It's often assumed by many that carbs' only job is to provide energy, and sure, it's true that your body breaks them down and turns them into stored short-term fuel in the form of simple sugars. However, carbohydrates also help the cells and molecules in your body talk to one another, acting as receptors so that cells can sense and recognize one another. In addition, carbs fortify cells by creating layers around them that offer support and protection.

Your body processes carbohydrates on three levels:

1. **It converts carbs into energy it can use immediately (glucose).** This type of sugar is released into your bloodstream 24/7 and is the fuel behind the everyday functions that keep you alive.
2. **It converts carbs into reserve energy it can use later (glycogen).** This version of glucose gets stored mostly in the liver (where it's used as fuel for your brain) and within your muscles (for deployment there).
3. Finally, **it converts carbs into back-up energy it might need eventually (body fat).**

How those carbohydrates get divvied up depends on the body consuming them. Priority goes to glucose so that the body maintains stores of immediate energy, but once those needs are met, carbohydrates begin to refill the stores of glycogen in the liver and muscles. Your body can only hold so much of that reserve energy, though, so if there are any additional calories floating around, it assumes you want to use them later and stores them as fat.

To make matters a little more confusing, not all carbohydrates are equal. They come in two versions—simple and complex. Simple carbs—like the kind you'll find in honey, corn syrup, sugar (both granulated and brown), molasses, and maple syrup, for example—earn their name because they're made from only one or two sugar molecules and lack many nutrients or fiber, which makes it effortless for your body to process them. Complex carbohydrates—typically found in whole plant foods such as vegetables, wheat, and rice, in addition to foods made from them (pasta, bread, etc.)—are, well, a little more complex. They're made from three or more sugar molecules and have more nutrients and fiber, which means your body needs to spend more time and effort to digest them.

You need to understand the difference between the two because it is complex carbohydrates that I'm urging you to eat at every meal. Most carb-rich foods out there contain simple carbs, and because they get processed so quickly, if that's all you eat, your body will always have more sugar floating around than your system needs. That sugar surge raises your body's blood glucose levels. Your body then releases excess insulin (a hormone that removes sugar from your blood and puts it into your cells where it can be metabolized for energy), causing those carbs to be stored as unwanted body fat. Do it too often and your body becomes less effective at lowering your blood sugar, so it releases even more insulin. Eventually, it can't keep up, so your blood sugar stays elevated, causing what is known as insulin resistance, a condition that is not only linked to both high blood sugar and obesity, but is the main cause of many health issues, including type-2 diabetes, cardiovascular disease, nonalcoholic fatty liver disease, and metabolic syndrome.

Ideally, you want to maintain a very low level of circulating sugar in your bloodstream. This will satisfy your energy needs without causing any sugar spikes that can trigger an insulin response. In other words, "eat like a bird—just enough to fly," giving your body what it immediately can use and never so much that it doesn't know what to do with it all. That's where complex carbohydrates come in. Because they are richer in vitamins and minerals and typically packed with fiber, they take much longer to digest, allowing your body to benefit from an advantage of a more consistent, steady stream of sugar. And they boast longevity benefits beyond that.

You see, fiber is a carbohydrate that the body can't break down—but that it desperately needs. Fiber comes in two forms: soluble and insoluble. Soluble fiber turns spongelike when it dissolves in water and moves through the digestive tract, assisting in stabilizing blood sugar levels by slowing down the absorption of carbohydrates. Insoluble fiber doesn't dissolve in water, so it helps clean the digestive track and keeps the body regular. Collectively, the two types of fiber are unquestionably a powerful tag team, shown by science to lower the odds of metabolic syndrome, obesity, cardiovascular disease, and diabetes,[1] and eating high amounts has proven to reduce the risk of coronary heart disease, stroke, type-2 diabetes, colorectal cancer, and all-cause and cardiovascular-related death by 15 to 31 percent.[2]

You would think with so much going for it that fiber would be the number one consideration most people would look for in their food, but it's not. The magic number that most doctors and dieticians agree we should be shooting for is between 25 and 30 grams of fiber a day, but sadly, statistics show that roughly 90 percent of Americans don't get there.[3] So, when I stress that I want to see each meal or snack have some form of complex carbohydrates present, know that every time you make the effort to have that happen, you're not just extending your longevity in terms of performance, but literally extending your life.

Final point: Some of the foods I'm going to recommend later in the book may seem like simple carbohydrates because of how rich they are in natural sugar. Think sweet fruits in particular: oranges, cherries, apples, and so forth. Technically, there are some fruits and vegetables made up of simple carbohydrates. However, because these fruits and vegetables also contain a certain amount of protein (it's often trace amounts, but it's there), soluble and insoluble fiber, and other nutrients, your body *treats them* like complex carbohydrates. Just know that whatever carbohydrates I'm recommending, they are essential for providing your body with just the right amount of energy.

Fats

Before I explain the importance of healthy fats in your diet, let's get one thing clear: The excess fat on your body that you might not be a fan of isn't the result of *eating* fat. Like I mentioned earlier when discussing carbohydrates, whatever you're not happy about fat-wise on your body is the result of eating more calories than your body required—it's as simple as that. *Body* fat has nothing to do with the type of fats found in your food. Those are *dietary* fats, and they come in four different types.

The Healthy Kinds

Monounsaturated fats (or MUFAs): Found in certain foods such as olives, avocados, and nuts—peanuts, almonds, cashews, and pecans, for example—as well as certain oils (canola, olive, peanut, sesame, sunflower, etc.), monounsaturated fats typically are liquid at room temperature but solid when kept below that temp. These are considered "healthy fats." Eating MUFA-rich foods has been shown to lower your LDL cholesterol levels (along with your chances of developing cardiovascular disease), and they can also reduce your risk of certain cancers and ease inflammation.

Polyunsaturated fats (or PUFAs): Found in fatty fish and seafood (tuna, salmon, herring, mackerel, shrimp, scallops, and sardines, for example), certain nuts and seeds (walnuts, chia, sunflower, pumpkin, etc.), and also in certain plant-based oils (canola, olive, sunflower, etc.), PUFAs also usually liquefy at room temperature and turn solid when cooled down. And, as you might expect, this healthy fat also promotes better health like MUFAs by lowering your risk of heart disease by improving your blood cholesterol levels. They also benefit your body in many other ways, including minimizing inflammation in your joints and reducing your risk of cancer. But where they bring a little extra to the playing field is by assisting with blood clotting, building cell membranes, and being fortified with two fatty acids that your body can't produce on its own but are essential for good health: omega-3 and omega-6 fatty acids. Omega-3s boost your immune system and benefit your neurons—the cells that transmit signals throughout your body to your brain.

The Unhealthy Kinds

Saturated fats: This type of fat—which comes mostly from higher-fat meats (such as beef, dark-meat chicken, lamb, and pork), egg yolks, cheese, butter, whole-fat dairy products, and certain processed foods—stays solid at room temperature. It's considered an unhealthy fat because of (among other reasons) how it elevates LDL cholesterol—the kind that raises your chances of developing cardiovascular disease—and may boost your risk of suffering from type-2 diabetes down the line.

Trans fats: This final version is found in some meat and dairy products, but for the most part this fat hides inside processed foods. It helps extend the shelf life of things like baked goods, packaged snacks, stick margarine, and a lot of fried fare. Just like saturated fats, trans fats raise bad cholesterol (LDL), but they go one step further by lowering your good cholesterol (HDL), which makes you even more likely to develop cardiovascular disease. Trans fats also boost your body's level of triglycerides, which can cause inflammation as well as thicken your artery walls, making you more likely to develop atherosclerosis.

NOW, ALL THAT SAID, YOU need fat in your diet. But when I say you should have a serving of "healthy fats" with each meal and snack, I'm talking about foods rich in monounsaturated and polyunsaturated fats. Because in addition to the heart-healthy, inflammation-easing perks of MUFAs and PUFAs, fat is a slow-burning energy source that, when paired with the right amount of complex carbohydrates and lean protein, will leave you feeling satiated for a longer period of time—making you less likely to reach for calories you don't need hours after you eat.

Water

You're probably familiar with the recommendation to drink 64 ounces of water, or eight 8-ounce glasses, each day. But I tell my clients to double that.

Sixteen glasses of water each day might seem like way too much, but if that's your initial reaction, I'm guessing you've never tried it. Maybe the reason is because you have no interest in going to the bathroom more often than usual. That part might be true, but the trade-off is that there's a few other things that increase as a result—your performance, muscle size and strength, overall endurance, and willpower when it comes to avoiding unhealthy foods.

Think about this: The human body can survive for weeks without food but only three days without water. Why is that? It's because literally every single cell in your body contains water—and every single function within your body requires it to do its job. Let that absorb (pardon the pun) for a second. How your body reacts, how efficiently it builds and maintains lean muscle, how able it is to access energy and utilize stored fat as fuel, how quickly it can heal itself and fight off infection—and the list goes on—whatever your body is trying to do, it needs water.

So doesn't it make sense that, if you're dehydrated right now, you are holding back everything your body is capable of? In fact, research has long proven that losing just 1 to 2 percent of your body weight in fluid can impair performance and adversely affect recovery by as much as 20 percent. If you weigh 175 pounds, that's just 28 to 56 ounces of water. Add the fact that being dehydrated not only leaves you feeling less satiated, but causes your body to crave water from wherever it can find it, which can lead to overeating.

The Rules of the Regimen

The rules are simple and worth repeating. Every meal or snack should contain:

- One serving of high-quality protein
- One serving of complex carbohydrates
- One serving of healthy fats
- A minimum of 8 to 12 ounces of water

[Note: If you're not sure what one serving of each looks like, I've provided a variety of charts starting on page 50 to help get you started.]

Now, how you follow these rules matters. A few tips:

Eat five or six small meals throughout the day, as opposed to having two or three large meals. That means breakfast, lunch, and dinner with a snack in between. Eating these smaller, complex meals that have a higher nutritional value provides the best bang for your buck for several reasons:

- You'll have a constant level of energy that keeps your blood sugar levels even all day, preventing the release of excess insulin (so you'll store less body fat) and any cravings for more calories than your body needs. Gone is that feeling of sluggishness at certain hours of the day.
- Your body will continuously have access to protein so that it always has what it needs to build and repair itself.
- You'll absorb more vitamins, minerals, amino acids, and other important nutrients since your body can only process so much at one time.

Have around 6 to 8 ounces of water on the half hour. You can sip it throughout those thirty minutes, or pound it back every time the minute hand strikes either :30 or :00. It's your choice, but I don't want you to trust your sense of thirst. Instead, I just want you to drink enough to keep your fluid levels high so that you're guaranteed to end the day having finished off a total of 1 gallon.

Score each meal/snack and tally things up at the end of the day. For each of the elements of any meal you manage to pull off—protein, complex carbs, healthy fats, and water—give yourself a point each, then see how you did at the end of the day. At a maximum 4 points possible for each meal/snack, the highest score you could get (depending on if you eat five or six times a day) would be either 20 or 24.

Now, that said, do I expect you to get a perfect score every day, every week, every month, and so forth for the rest of your life? C'mon now.

Nobody has landed every punch, struck out every batter, or caught every pass. So why would I expect you to stick the landing at every meal or snack? Truth be told, no one is capable of that, and the goal here is not perfectionism, it's sustainability. Our goal together is to make solid and sound decisions that will positively affect your long-term health and performance. Trust me, I get that with sustainability comes volatility.

See, as much as this program is about longevity and prolonging performance, trying to adhere to that kind of "impossible perfection" doesn't hold any value. Life is all about balance, and enjoying something unhealthy occasionally may not be the best thing for us nutritionally, but it can sometimes bring a form of comfort that balances us in ways that nothing else can. So what I want you to do is what every athlete does: I want you to aim for perfection and try your absolute best with each meal, then use that score as a guide to instantly assess how you're doing that day. But if you don't stick the landing, don't use that score to beat yourself up. Instead, build yourself up by using it as motivation to do better at the next meal.

Final Things to Note

Now as I've stressed, this isn't a typical diet—it's just a set of general guidelines that point the way of *how* to eat. Which foods you choose to fill each role is entirely up to you. But before you start, I urge you to keep the following things in mind:

Keep it light. For now, try to keep your meals to just one serving each of protein, carbs, and fats and 8 to 12 ounces of water. See how it makes you feel. Could your body acquire a little more calorically? Possibly, but you might be surprised at how satiated you are, how much more energy you have, and how much better you feel eating what most likely is less than you typically might at a sitting.

Keep it clean. Whatever sources you choose, I want you to reach for the cleanest, freshest foods as often as possible. The fewer artificial additives you ingest—fillers, chemicals, and other unnatural ingredients—the more benefits you'll get from every meal, whether you can see or feel their impact on your body or not. So if you have the chance to eat wild game or fish, free-range chicken, grass-fed beef, or pasture-raised pork instead of conventionally produced meat or fish that may be pumped full of hormones and antibiotics, take it. That same attention to production methods also goes for fruits, vegetables, and just about anything else.

Keep it on track. Listen, I know trying to hit these numbers as often as possible might seem like a chore, but it really doesn't take any more time than other tasks connected to what we eat when you think about it. We have no problem spending a few minutes figuring out what to eat based on what we're in the mood for, how many calories it has, or the price on the menu. Is it really that painful or difficult to use that same amount of time looking at a meal's nutritional content from a performance and longevity standpoint? Get in the habit of giving every meal or snack a quick once-over so you feel confident that what you're seconds away from throwing back is going to move your body forward.

Keep it real. Am I saying to never choose anything based on taste, even if it is high in calories and low in nutrients? Absolutely not. Food is to be enjoyed and I would never deny you the satisfaction of sitting down with a great meal, no matter how bad it might be for you. But the more you understand what you're eating—an education that comes from taking the time to think about what's within every item of food before you eat it—the more likely you'll be to make better food choices more often after you've polished off that unhealthy treat.

The Charts to Give You a Head Start

Beyond the basics I've just explained to you, what you choose in terms of protein, complex carbohydrates, and healthy fats each meal or snack is entirely up to you. To make what you pick and choose a little easier, I've listed a variety of foods you can easily combine. Just remember the following:

1. Certain foods technically help you pull off a twofer (meaning, one serving might check off more than one box when it comes to getting a serving of protein, carbohydrates, and fats). For example, fatty fish and certain seafood such as tuna, herring, mackerel, and even anchovies are all rich sources of protein, but they're also abundant in healthy fats. Nuts are rich in healthy fats, but they're also a complex carbohydrate. You can choose to check off two boxes if you like (and see the same food on two different charts) or opt to cover your bases and stick with eating three different types of foods in each meal or snack.
2. I've kept these portion sizes at the low end in terms of average serving sizes. Chances are you may eat an ounce (or even two) more of a particular source, and that's fine. I don't want you to be so concerned with the fine print that it keeps you from being excited about eating healthier. Even though I've listed the caloric amounts of each food within this chart, it's meant more as a reference than as a strict rule.
3. Within the list of complex carbohydrates, are some more, shall we say, "complex" than others? Absolutely. Depending on which food you choose, how slowly your body will break down that food will depend on its nutritional makeup. Even if you choose, for example, a piece of fruit with a high sugar content and less fiber than other fruits or vegetables, one that may not rank high on the "complex carbohydrate" list of major achievers, it still beats reaching for simple carbohydrates as an energy source.
4. Finally, don't expect to see everything in here. Listing every possible source would take up more real estate than necessary. Use these charts as guides, but I encourage you to explore other options beyond them once you get familiar with the formula.

Some Quality Protein Options

Food	Portion Size	Protein (gm)	Carbs (gm)	Total Fat (gm)	Saturated fat (gm)	Calories
Anchovies (drained)	One 2-oz. can	13	0	4	1	94
Atlantic cod (baked)	3 oz.	19	0	1	0	89
Atlantic herring (baked)	3 oz.	20	0	10	2	172
Atlantic mackerel (baked)	3 oz.	21	0	16	4	230
Beef tenderloin (lean, boneless, and roasted)	3 oz.	24	0	6	2	152
Bison (roasted)	3 oz.	24	0	2	1	123

Bluefish (baked)	3 oz.	22	0	5	1	135
Bottom round (lean and cooked)	3 oz.	24	0	5	2	139
Brisket (lean and braised)	3 oz.	28	0	6	2	174
Brown trout (baked)	3 oz.	22	0	3	2	119
Canadian bacon	3 oz.	21	0	6	3	156
Carp (baked)	3 oz.	19	0	6	1	138
Catfish (steamed)	3 oz.	17	0	8	2	144

Chicken breast (boneless)	3 oz.	25	0	3	1	128
Chicken breast (with bone)	3 oz.	25	0	7	2	168
Chicken thigh (boneless)	3 oz.	21	0	8	2	166
Chicken thigh (with bone)	3 oz.	15	0	9	3	149
Chuck roast (lean and braised)	3 oz.	28	0	6	2	179
Cobia	3 oz.	16	2.5	5.5	1.8	125
Cottage cheese (nonfat)	4 oz.	11	7	0	0	80

Duck breast (broiled)	3 oz.	23	0	2	0	119
Egg (whole)	1 large	6	0	5	2	70
Egg white	1 large	4	0	0	0	17
Eye round (lean and roasted)	3 oz.	25	0	3	1	138
Filet mignon (lean and broiled)	3 oz.	24	0	9	3	179
Flank steak (lean and braised)	3 oz.	23	0	14	6	224
Flank steak (lean and broiled)	3 oz.	24	0	6	3	158

Flounder (baked)	3 oz.	21	0	1	0	100
Ground beef (70% lean/30% fat)	3 oz.	12	0	25	9.5	279
Ground beef (80% lean/20% fat)	3 oz.	14	0	17	6.5	213
Ground beef (extra lean)	3 oz.	22	0	13	5	208
Grouper (baked)	3 oz.	21	0	1	0	100
Haddock (baked or steamed)	3 oz.	21	0	1	0	95
Halibut (baked)	3 oz.	23	0	3	0	119

Jerky (beef)	1 oz.	9.5	3	7	3	116
Jerky (turkey)	1 oz.	15	3	.5	0	80
Lamb chop (lean and broiled)	3 oz.	26	0	8	3	184
Mahi-mahi (baked)	3 oz.	20	0	1	0	93
Milk (whole)	1 cup	8	11.5	5	3	122
Milk (1%)	1 cup	8	12	2	1.5	102
Milk (nonfat)	1 cup	8	12	.5	.25	86

Orange roughy (baked)	3 oz.	19	0	1	0	89
Ostrich (ground)	3 oz.	22	0	6	2	149
Pheasant	3 oz.	28	0	10	3	210
Pork tenderloin (roasted)	3 oz.	24	0	4	1	139
Rib steak (lean and broiled)	3 oz.	12	0	3	1	81
Roast beef (lunch meat)	3 oz.	18	3	3	3	90
Salmon (baked or broiled)	3 oz.	17	0	5	1	118

Sardines	One 3.75-oz. can	23	0	11	1	191
Scallops (steamed or broiled)	5	10	2	2	0	70
Sea bass (baked)	3 oz.	20	0	2	1	105
Shrimp	3 oz.	20	1	1.5	.5	100
Sole (baked)	3 oz.	21	0	1	0	100
Striped bass (baked)	3 oz.	19	0	3	1	105
T-Bone (lean and broiled)	3 oz.	22	0	8	3	168

Top round steak (braised)	3 oz.	30	0	5	2	178
Top sirloin steak (broiled)	3 oz.	26	0	6	2	166
Tuna (bluefin; baked)	3 oz.	25	0	5	1	156
Tuna (canned, in water)	3 oz.	20	0	3	1	109
Turkey breast (roasted with skin)	3 oz.	24	0	6	2	161
Turkey dark meat (roasted with skin)	3 oz.	23	0	10	3	188
Turkey leg	3 oz.	24	0	8	3	177

Veal chop (lean and braised)	3 oz.	29	0	8	2	192
Venison	3 oz.	25	0	8	2	177
Whitefish	3 oz.	21	0	6	1	146
Yogurt (plain, low-fat)	8 oz.	12	16	3.5	2	143
Yogurt (plain, nonfat)	8 oz.	13	17	.5	.26	127

Some Complex Carbohydrate Options

Food	Portion Size	Protein (gm)	Carbs (gm)	Fat (gm)	Calories
Acorn squash	½ cup	1	15	0	57
Apple	1	0	19	0	72
Apricot (fresh)	2 or 3	0	5	0	20
Artichoke (small)	1	3	10	0	50
Asparagus	4 oz.	3	5	0	25
Banana (8 inches)	1	1	31	0	121
Beets (cooked)	⅓ cup	1	6	0	24
Blackberries	½ cup	1	7	.5	31
Black beans	½ cup	7.6	20	.5	113
Blueberries	½ cup	1	11	0	41
Broccoli (steamed)	½ cup	2	4	0	22
Brussels sprouts	1 cup	4	11	1	56

Bulgur (cooked)	1 cup	6	34	.4	151
Butternut squash (baked)	½ cup	1	11	0	41
Cabbage (chopped)	½ cup	.5	3	0	11
Cantaloupe	½ cup	.5	7	0	13
Carrot (medium size)	1	.5	3	0	13
Cauliflower	½ cup	1	3	0	15
Celery stalks (large)	2	0	4	0	20
Cherries (sour)	½ cup	1	9	0	39
Chickpeas (garbanzo beans)	½ cup	7.3	22.5	2	134
Corn (sweet yellow)	⅓ cup	1	10	0	41
Couscous (cooked)	⅓ cup	2	12	0	59
Edamame	½ cup	11	10	6	127
Eggplant	1 cup	1	9	0	35

Ezekiel sprouted grain bread	1 slice	4	15	1	80
Grapefruit (medium size)	1	2	20	0	82
Grapes (green or red)	½ cup	1	14	0	55
Green beans	½ cup	1	4	0	19
Kidney beans	½ cup	7.7	20	.4	112
Lentils	½ cup	9	20	.4	115
Lima beans	½ cup	7.3	21	.3	115
Mango	1	2	36	0	134
Nectarine (medium size)	1	1	17	0	70
Oats (regular or instant)	½ cup	5.3	27.4	2.6	153
Oats (steel-cut)	¼ cup	5	27	2.5	150
Orange (medium size)	1	1	16	0	66
Papaya	1 cup	1	14	0	52
Peach (medium size)	1	1	9	0	38

Pear (medium size)	1	1	26	0	100
Peas	½ cup	4	10	4	59
Pineapple	1 cup	1	22	0	82
Pinto beans	½ cup	8	22	.6	122
Pita (whole wheat)	1	6	36	2	170
Plum (medium size)	1	0	8	0	30
Portobello mushroom	1 cup	2	4	0	22
Potato (medium size, baked with skin)	1	4	36	0	162
Prunes (medium size)	3	1	13	0	50
Pumpernickel bread	1 slice	2	12	1	65
Quinoa (cooked)	⅓ cup	4	20	1	108
Raspberries	½ cup	.5	8	0	32
Rice (basmati)	½ cup	3	35	0	162
Rice (brown, medium, or long-grain)	⅓ cup	1.5	15	0	72

Rye bread	1 slice	3	15	1	82
Seven-grain bread	1 slice	3	12	1	65
Snow peas (steamed)	½ cup	2	6	0	35
Spinach (cooked)	½ cup	2.5	3.5	0	20
Strawberries	½ cup	.5	7	0	26
Summer squash (baked)	½ cup	1	11	0	41
Sweet potato (peeled, cooked, and mashed)	½ cup	2	29	0	125
Tomato (medium size)	1	1	7	1	35
Whole-wheat bread	1 slice	3	13	1	69
Whole-wheat pasta	1 cup	7.6	38	1	176
Yams (cooked)	½ cup	2	18	0	78
Zucchini (steamed)	½ cup	1	3	0	13

Some Healthy Fat Options

Food	Portion Size	Protein (gm)	Carbs (gm)	Fat (gm)	Saturated Fat (gm)	Calories
Almond butter	1 tbsp.	3	3	9	1	102
Almonds	1 oz.	6	6	14	1	164
Anchovies (drained)	One 2-oz. can	13	0	4	1	94
Atlantic herring (baked)	3 oz.	20	0	10	2	172
Atlantic mackerel (baked)	3 oz.	21	0	16	4	230
Avocado	½ cup	2	6	10	2	116
Bluefish (baked)	3 oz.	22	0	5	1	135

Butter	1 tsp.	0	0	4	2	33
Brazil nuts	1 oz.	4	3.5	19	4	186
Cashew butter	1 tbsp.	3	5	10	2	110
Cashew nuts	1 oz.	5	9	14	2.4	165
Chestnuts (roasted)	1 oz.	1	15	1	0	69
Chia seeds	1 oz.	4.4	12.4	8.7	1	139
Cobia	3 oz.	16	2.5	5.5	1.8	125
Fish oil (cod liver, salmon, herring, or sardine)	1 tsp.	0	0	4.5	1	41

Flaxseeds (whole)	1 tbsp.	2	3	4	0	55
Macadamia nuts	1 oz.	2	4	21.5	3.5	204
Olive oil	1 tsp.	0	0	5	1	40
Olives (small)	14	.5	2.5	5	.5	53
Peanuts	1 oz.	7	4.5	14	2	161
Pecans	1 oz.	2.5	4	20.5	2	196
Pumpkin seeds (raw)	1 tbsp.	3	1	5	1	63
Salmon (baked or broiled)	3 oz.	17	0	5	1	118

Sardines	One 3.75-oz. can	23	0	11	1	191
Sesame seeds (roasted)	1 tbsp.	2	2	5	0	52
Striped bass (baked)	3 oz.	19	0	3	1	105
Sunflower seeds	1 oz.	6.5	5	14	1.5	162
Walnuts	1 oz.	4	4	18.5	2	185
Whitefish	3 oz.	21	0	6	1	146

CHAPTER 5

Break It Down

It doesn't matter what you take on in life—whether it's a sport, a job, a hobby, or anything that requires effort—I know this much: Even if you're the best at it, no one ever does anything perfectly, and no one ever does anything totally wrong.

As I brought up in the last chapter, eating healthy is one of those areas that nobody gets right 100 percent of the time. There are moments of perfection in the worst performances, just as there are mistakes made by those that come out on top. Whenever we try to achieve something, no matter what it is, there are portions of our performance where we excel and other portions where we trip up.

That's normal, that's life, and that's you. That's me too and every single person on the planet. Most decisions about food will contain both good and bad elements. You can either choose to obsess over the bad ones—or you can learn from them.

Once you finish eating, the thought of food typically doesn't enter your mind until the next meal—but that's a huge mistake. Instead, before you step away from the table, you need to assess the nutritional choices you just made in that moment and concentrate on what your body is trying to tell you.

Now, I know what you're thinking: "But, Mike—I really don't have time to do this every time I eat!" First off, there is always time. How many times have you finished a meal and found yourself sitting there at the table socializing long after you cleaned off your plate?

I'll give you that there will be moments immediately after a meal or snack that you might not be able to do what I'm asking you to—if you're eating on the go, for example, or have to go right back to work after lunch. But the minutes are always there during the day at some point. Besides, all I'm insisting you do is run through a quick series of questions that'll take you a couple minutes at most, writing your answers on a piece of paper or in your phone so you can easily refer to them later.

If you think that it's easier to reflect on everything you ate during the day at the *end* of the day, then you're cheating yourself of one of the benefits of doing it sequentially. Because the way each meal affects you will shift over the course of several hours, and it's important to chart that progression. Let's break it down:

1. How Do You Feel Now Compared to Then?

Remember when I had you reflect on four questions right before you ate?

1. Where would you rank your hunger?
2. Where would you rank your thirst?
3. Where would you rank your energy level?
4. Where would you rank your stress level?

After eating, I want you to ask yourself how you would rank each question again to look for any significant changes.

Hunger: That number should be lower than it was, but if it's not a 1, don't be too concerned. It's okay to feel a little hungry after a meal. You should feel satisfied and light—and never stuffed. The object isn't to leave the table so full that even thinking of taking another bite would be impossible. Instead, it's about asking yourself, "Do I feel satisfied to wait two to three hours until my next meal?"

Thirst: This number *should* be a 1, so if it's not quite there before you step away from the table, you need to get it there.

Energy: This one is tricky, because the moment you eat, your body begins to direct a certain portion of its energy toward digestion, which can leave you feeling a little more tired than when you started. However, that's where eating smaller, more frequent meals should help. The fewer calories your body has to break down afterward, the more energized you will feel. Ideally, you should feel satisfied (not sluggish) and slightly more alert.

Stress: This one may be the most important of the four, so really consider whether that number went up, went down, or even stayed the same, because:

- **If it's lower**—was it because you weren't sure you could pull off eating healthy at that moment and felt proud that you did? Did sitting there give you time to contemplate or solve whatever was stressing you out in the first place? Or did just pausing for a few minutes for a meal give you enough of a breather to unwind? I won't know why you feel less stressed, so it's worth taking a moment to figure it out so that you might take advantage of that knowledge at the next meal.
- **If it's higher**—was it because you were using eating to avoid facing whatever was stressing you out? Or because you were running late for something and it took you longer than expected to eat, so you're even further behind?
- **If it's the same**—then if your number was high to begin with (yet didn't budge), use this meal as a reminder that turning to food when stressed doesn't change whatever it is you're concerned about. That's an important lesson to learn because so many of us reach for comfort food (aka crap) as an escape from what's really bothering us. Meanwhile, it just creates new problems by affecting our health, our self-esteem, and our performance.

Because I'm asking you to eat every two or three hours, I want you to revisit these questions a second time roughly sixty to ninety minutes after you've eaten. The effects of what we eat aren't always felt immediately. If you touch base with yourself at this midpoint between meals, you'll come to recognize the impact of eating a more balanced, performance-driven meal.

2. What Took It to the Next Level?

Whatever you chose to eat was just that—a choice. If you made the right one, a question remains: What made you choose to eat the best foods for your body at that meal? I mean, I might've told you what to eat, but you made a conscious choice to do it. What exactly made it *just a little bit easier* to find that willpower?

This is something many people never think about. We'll pick apart why we might have eaten *poorly* and blame it on this or that. (Don't worry, we'll be doing that in a second.) And occasionally, we might even give ourselves a pat on the back for eating wisely as well. Yet very few people ever stop to consider what might've helped them eat wisely. But that's exactly what I want you to do.

Awareness: Truth be told, the more you understand why certain foods are healthy for you and others are not, the harder it becomes to ignore the right way to eat. So did you choose a certain food because you were knowledgeable about how healthy it was, what types of nutrients were inside it, or how it fuels your body in a more efficient way? If knowing about a food's benefits is the reason you chose it, then begin taking the time to learn more about other healthier choices you could be making as well.

Preparation: Most of us are crunched for time, and whatever is easiest to reach for is typically what makes it onto our plates. So did you do anything differently to make healthier foods more accessible? If planning ahead is partly responsible for you staying the course, then I urge you to continue doing that, but also explore other ways you could be making things a little easier for yourself in the future.

Maybe you've noticed that you seem to make smarter choices when you wake up a half hour earlier. Or did you plan ahead and prepare a week's worth of grilled chicken or make a huge bowl of sliced fruit you could reach for in a pinch? Did you discover that your local supermarket has an entire section of "at the ready" meals that fit the requirements I'm hoping you'll stick to? Whatever decisions helped you make smarter nutritional choices, it's time to consider doubling down and making them a bigger part of your routine.

Those around you: The people who surround you *when* you eat can play a huge part in *what* you eat. In this case, having like-minded, health-conscious people at the table can make it less stressful to be particular about what you choose to consume. Was that the case? Did knowing that you wouldn't be critiqued or judged ease the sting? Or was it because the person you were dining across from or throwing back food in the car with is one of your "rocks" and they're fully aware of what you're trying to achieve? In any case, if support from your people was part of your success, then invite them over (or out) for meals often, or ask if it's all right to check in with them (via text, phone call, or FaceTime) for a little encouragement right before a meal when you feel you might be more inclined to eat poorly.

Curiosity: Maybe you discovered a new protein drink or finally decided to try a particular fruit or vegetable simply because you had never had it before. Curiosity may have killed a few cats as they say, but when it comes to eating for longevity, exploration can revive your enthusiasm. If wondering about something healthy—whether it's how it tastes, what its texture is like, how it's prepared, whatever—is what managed to put that good-for-you option on your plate, then take a few minutes each day to research other fruits, vegetables, protein sources, nuts, seeds (you name it!) that you've always been curious about. That way, you'll be more likely to repeat that same success, while at the same time expanding your horizons when it comes to your palette.

Looking for a little inspirational help? Start with the obvious by going to your supermarket and making a list of any fruits, vegetables, and other healthy fare you've never tried before or haven't had in a long time. I've also found that visiting local farmer's stands and ethnic markets is a great way to encounter people who not only can point you in the direction of foods you never knew existed, but even offer advice on different ways to prepare them.

Atmosphere: For some people, simply changing the scenery can be a tremendous motivating force toward eating better. It could be eating somewhere entirely different that helps you avoid seeing or being exposed to unhealthy foods. Maybe taking your lunch outside and being at one with nature gave you inspiration? Or choosing to sit down at a table to eat instead of grabbing a meal on the go and tossing it down in your car was a deciding factor? Ask yourself if the environment you surrounded yourself with had a hand in any way, and if so, do your best to hang out there as often as possible.

3. What Stood in the Way of Success?

Before I have you break anything down—and you should expect to hear this type of frank talk later in this book when I ask you to do the same with how you're moving and mending—I don't want you wasting a single second dumping on yourself or wishing you could've done even better. Because for a lot of people, that attitude can sometimes lead to repeated failure. Dwell too much on how you blew your diet during one meal and you can beat yourself up to the point that you assume you'll never be able to eat healthy on a consistent basis—so you quit altogether.

You screwed up—so what? We all screw up, and whatever junk food, cholesterol-packed meal, or fat-laced condiment you doused on top of it all—every single thing that didn't have any nutritional value whatsoever—is literally being eaten by somebody else right now as you read this. And if we're really being honest here, it's something that even the greatest of athletes sneak into their diet occasionally. LeBron is right up there for having chocolate-chip cookies as his kryptonite. Whether we like it or not, willpower when it comes to what we eat and drink sort of ebbs and flows, depending on the kind of day we're having. But that doesn't mean you can't steer it in the direction you need it to go.

It's no different from having a bad day at work, a bad moment with your partner, or a bad game at whatever sport you enjoy. This is the entire point of breaking things down *after* the fact. By addressing each mistake—and that's all each one is, just a simple mistake—it lets you acknowledge that, okay, you made a less than optimal choice in that moment. Who cares? It proves you're human. Now, let's figure out why it happened so that we can minimize or possibly eliminate the chance of it happening the next time you're in a similar situation.

Lack of time: Let's begin with the most common excuse for making poor dietary choices. Most of us feel like we have barely enough minutes in the day as it is, so being told to spend time on food prep before each meal can be a big ask—and I get that. But the fact is, if life is busy now for you *today*, then I hate to break it to you, but it's not going to be any less busy for you tomorrow. That's why putting an end to this obstacle as soon as possible should be job number one.

Is that you? There's no blame or shame here, but if lack of time caused you to veer off course, then let's think about how to prevent that from happening again:

- **Look for the wasted minutes.** First, you need to take a hard and honest look at how you're spending your time. If that takes literally breaking down what you're doing every five minutes of your day from the time your eyes open in the morning until the time they close at night to fall asleep, I suggest you do it because I've never met anyone who filled their entire day with important tasks. Even high performers waste plenty of time that can be redirected toward making smart choices. Find your stolen minutes—even if it's just a few—then aim them toward food preparation instead.
- **Retrace your steps.** Was the situation that kept you from eating healthier completely avoidable if you had planned better? For example, if getting up at the same time as your kids on a school morning leaves you little time for yourself because you're too busy getting them ready and out the door, then set your clock earlier. Point being, if it's ever a question of not having enough time to plan, then figure out what or who stole time

away from you and ask yourself how you can prevent that from happening again (or at least occurring as often), then take action.

Obligation: We've all been put in positions in which we ate or drank things we didn't want but felt obligated to, because we either didn't want to offend someone or didn't want to be the odd man out.

Is that you? Then question yourself why you couldn't say no. I mean, really run through the scenario by picturing the outcome if you had just said, "Hey, you know what? I'm trying to eat a little better for health reasons, so if it's okay with you, I'm going to pass for now, but thank you." Chances are the response won't be severe or negative—in fact, it's likely to be encouraging! And if it *is* negative—if someone you're with would be that put off by what you're trying to do for yourself—then that's not a rock you can count on.

Now, I understand that it could be a work situation, wedding, or party where you may not want to stand out so much. Or it could be a friend, spouse, significant other, or relative who really wants you to try that high-caloric, pure-sugar dessert they just whipped up, and turning them down would break their heart. In those instances, they typically are one-off situations that you shouldn't beat yourself up for indulging. However, if these "every once in a while" moments happen a little too frequently, then it's time to either figure out a way to best avoid them or muster up the courage to explain why you can't indulge as often.

Tension: Even if "stress" didn't score high on your list when I asked you to rate your stress level both before and after you ate, just having "a little bit on your mind" before a meal can take you down a different path.

Is that you? Trying to tell yourself to get to the bottom of whatever's stressing you out is the obvious solution, but that's not always possible. You could be going through something that's not easily solved in a day, week, or month—heck, it might not even be within your power to change—and if that describes your situation, I'm sorry to hear that. But if that's truly the case, and stress is negatively impacting your ability to eat healthy on a regular basis, then you need to figure out a way to separate your eating habits from your personal or professional dilemmas.

With clients, I'll advise them to try a variety of nonfood-based methods that have been shown to disconnect the two, such as jotting down in a journal whatever's stressing them out, as well as taking a ten-minute walk (even if it's pacing within their own house) whenever they find themselves reaching for food. Either act is usually enough to keep your brain busy and your body out of the kitchen. Fortunately, some of the techniques within the Mend section of the book will help alleviate many symptoms of stress, but not turning to food when stressed (particularly poorer nutritional choices) or allowing stress to interfere in any way with your ability to regularly pull together healthier meals should be your top priority.

Temptation: Cravings can be a powerful thing. Often they can feel impossible to deny—but that doesn't mean you can't. Don't get me wrong, sometimes we all just feel like eating bad. It's undeniable that there's a certain satisfaction from cheating on our diets, even if that bliss is fleeting. But if you let it happen too often—more important, if you don't understand why you're having those cravings in the first place—it can be a habit that's hard to break, and that will only make the longevity goals you have for yourself harder to obtain.

Reflect back on when you satisfied that craving. You may come to realize that what you've chosen as your "guilty pleasure" was picked for a reason that may be valid, but that doesn't mean it has to be unhealthy. In fact, it might not be about the ingredients of the foods you're eating, but the environment and emotions connected with that cheat meal that makes it hard to resist, such as:

- **Was it for the taste, texture, or temperature?** Meaning, were you craving something salty, sweet, or sour? Something crunchy or smooth? Hot or cold? Was that lemon meringue pie impossible to resist simply because you were in the mood for something lemony? Try to drill down into the "why" of what might've caused that craving in the first place, then consider if there are other ways you could've satisfied that urge with a healthier food that shares the same taste, texture, or temperature.

- **Was it out of routine?** When was the last time you felt the need to buy a basketball-sized tub of buttered popcorn outside of going to the movies? Right. Probably never—and that's the thing. Sometimes, the ties we have with bad food choices—decisions we otherwise would never go out of our way to make—are simply attached to habit.
- **Was it for nostalgia?** Sometimes we turn to foods that remind us of days gone by. I mean, it's hard not to forget you were ten once while chowing down on a bowl of sugary cereal, am I right? But if that's the reason you gave in to that specific craving—for the memory its taste or texture evoked—then you may need to explore other ways to achieve that same effect, such as listening to music or watching a television show on YouTube from that period of time, reminiscing with an old friend, or going through some things you've put away from back when.

NOW NOT ONLY DO YOU know, for better or for worse, what you did right or wrong when it comes to your meal—you're wiser as to why you made those decisions in the first place. Ready to put the pieces back together regarding what you put on your plate to make it easier to eat healthier? Then follow me!

CHAPTER 6

Rebuild It Better

Once you've owned what went wrong about a meal and recognized what went right, it's time to rethink ways to both minimize the chances of the same mistakes sabotaging your efforts and maximize your odds of repeating the same successes the next time you reach for something to eat. Just do me a favor as you begin to rebuild, and that's keep the following things in mind:

Hunger

Tell somebody to eat five to six times a day and they typically start at breakfast, enjoy a snack in between breakfast and lunch, have another snack in between lunch and dinner, then (if they're eating six times a day) have a snack a few hours after dinner. But putting some thought into the timing of when you start eating can help your body heal more efficiently.

As soon as you wake up—eat immediately! By the time you open your eyes, your body has already exhausted its stores of glycogen from fasting for the last six to eight hours, which leaves it little choice but to look for energy elsewhere. The problem is, your body really doesn't care where it finds that energy because it's in a catabolic state, so it starts breaking down—well, you! And as much as you'd like to think its first choice is stored fat, it's also tearing down lean muscle tissue right along with it. Ideally, before you even begin to even think about your day, you should get something in your stomach to pull your body out of panic mode.

Now, I entirely understand if preparing breakfast right out of bed isn't possible, but that's where your first snack comes in. Just tossing back a small snack can be just enough to trigger a hormonal response and release leptin, which can put a stop to that internal cannibalism immediately. That snack doesn't need to be huge to have a huge effect. Something as small as a half of a whole-wheat bagel topped with almond butter or a small banana and a handful of walnuts can keep your body from breaking itself down, plus meet that nutrient trifecta. (Say it with me again: *protein, complex carbohydrates, healthy fats.*)

Make yourself intentionally miss a meal. Why would I have you do this if everything I've stressed up until this point is to eat every two to three hours? Personal experimentation is good. I'm not saying to do this when you have a lot going on. Pick a day in which if your energy levels are off, it would not be the end of the world. Then purposely avoid eating a meal or snack so that you're waiting a good four to five hours in between—and really assess how you feel when that next meal finally comes.

See, chances are you're sometimes going to skip meals down the road. Usually, that's because the day got away from you, which means you probably have more on your mind than normal. Practicing skipping with purpose—when you aren't rushed or have other things to concern yourself with—helps build a better bond with your body's nutritional needs and demands. When you finally do eat on this test day, you should still run through the four questions I'm asking you to do at every meal: how would you rank your hunger, thirst, energy, and stress. But this time, I want you to look at how those numbers are different compared to usual. Notice how much hungrier or thirstier you are, if your energy is lower than usual, and, yes—even though I'm asking you to try this experiment on a more relaxed day—if you are a little more stressed out. It's a simple sacrifice, but one that connects you with the importance of purposely eating at the specific moments I'm asking you to by showing you the negative effects that can occur by doing otherwise.

Hydration

For some clients, just finding the time to drink a gallon of water every day is the greatest challenge, but as I mentioned earlier, it's literally worth every ounce. In fact, according to a new thirty-year study[1] by the National Institutes of Health involving over eleven thousand subjects, adults who stay hydrated not only develop fewer chronic conditions—including lung and heart disease—they live longer. Those who were less hydrated showed signs of faster biological aging, as well as a 21 percent increased risk of premature death. If that doesn't make it worth the extra few bathroom trips, I don't know what else will convince you. Here are a few tricks to make staying hydrated a little more manageable:

The earlier you sip, the better. It's been shown that healthy adults can process between 27 to 34 ounces of liquid per hour (going beyond that can lead to overhydration, which can overwork your kidneys and disrupt the ratio of electrolytes and fluids in your bloodstream). So the moment you wake up, start drinking. I encourage you to put a 12-ounce glass of water on your nightstand when you go to bed so you can polish it off before you even leave the bedroom—do that and you're already 10 percent of the way to your goal.

Plan out when it's easier to pee. Look, there are times during the day when the last thing you want to deal with is a full bladder. Plan ahead! If you know you have a forty-five-minute commute with no bathroom to be found, maybe you shouldn't chug a full bottle of water an hour before you leave. Strategically consider pockets of time when you know it will be either easier or more difficult for you to hit the head, then either raise or lower how much you're drinking roughly an hour (on average) ahead of time. Is it an exact science? Not at all, since each body is different in how quickly fluid moves through it. But simply applying common sense by asking yourself where you'll be in an hour as you drink should help you determine whether to save more of your sips for later or gulp down the lion's share at that moment.

When active, use the "fifteen-minute" rule. During exercise, sports, physical labor, or any moderately intense activity, you should drink about

16 to 32 ounces of water prior to that activity, then replenish with another 6 to 8 ounces every fifteen minutes. Making sure you stay hydrated lowers your risk of muscle cramps, speeds up your muscle's recovery time, keeps your energy levels high, and makes it easier for your heart to circulate blood throughout your body.

By the way, water is perfectly fine instead of electrolyte replacement drinks if you're active less than sixty minutes. However, if you go over an hour, switch to a sports drink instead with some form of carbohydrates in it for energy (nothing sugar-free or noncaloric). After that amount of time, your body will have burned through most of its stored glycogen, as well as lost through sweat a significant amount of sodium, potassium, and other electrolytes.

Amplify Your Accomplishments

I don't want you to settle for what took your diet to the next level—I want you to build on it. It's about taking every win, every moment of victory from your previous meals, and using them not only as examples to help motivate you during the next meal, but as opportunities to challenge yourself to take your nutrition a step further.

Amplify your awareness. If I told you research[2] has shown that your risk of all-cause mortality decreases by 12 percent for every 50 cents extra you spend daily on vegetables, would it motivate you to eat more vegetables? Could that be enough to make you less likely to skimp with that serving of salad?

Being educated on a topic can be incredibly inspiring, especially when it comes to matters of health. And if that's you—if knowing more details about the healthy foods I'm encouraging you to eat somehow makes the process a little easier to pull off during meals—then it's time to bone up. I'm talking about grabbing your phone right before or after you eat and looking up at least one thing about the food in front of you. It doesn't matter whether the food is healthy or unhealthy, so long as you do at least one of the following:

- **Learn one thing that's new.** Conducting medical studies takes time, but reading the results of the research doesn't have to. Being in the know as to why something is either healthy for you or not can be highly motivational, and it doesn't require a degree to do a little research. There are thousands of studies out there. All it takes is logging on to a search engine, typing in the kind of meat, fruit, vegetable, or whatever the food might be, then throwing in the word *research* or *study*, adding the current year, and seeing what pops up.
- **Learn one good thing.** If you're researching a healthy food, ask yourself first why you think it's healthy, then challenge yourself to find yet another reason it's good for you that you didn't know. The more you do this, the more you'll begin to pile on even more reasons why what you're eating is so vital for longevity.
- **Learn one bad thing.** The same rule applies if you're looking up something that's unhealthy that you're considering eating or already made the mistake of finishing off. Again, remind yourself what you know about it—what makes it bad for you—but try to find even more proof why that particular food should never be on your plate.

Final point: We all know that some research findings out there are supported by physicians, medical researchers, and companies who may have their own agendas, so how can you tell which studies are reputable? I admit that information can be hard to navigate, but here's the thing: I'm just suggesting that you learn a little bit more about why a particular healthy food is good for you and why a certain unhealthy food is bad for you. This is more of an exercise of exploration, and it's my hope that it makes you more curious about the foods you're being told to eat more of, as well as the ones you should avoid.

Amplify your preparation. Whenever you're out of your natural element—whether it's because you're traveling for work, vacationing, or scrambling to get to your kid's basketball game—it can be difficult to eat the way you should. Not having healthier options at your fingertips like you might at home can be a convenient excuse not to seek out healthier options elsewhere—but they *do* (or at least *can*) exist. It just takes a little extra work on your part.

The only way to always have the best foods at your fingertips is to plan ahead—something I know all too well. For me, constantly being on the road with LeBron means after I've booked where I'll be staying, the real work begins. For a lot of people, once that reservation's made, they might take that extra step and plan where they'll eat on certain days, but most never really take it any further than that. I do, not just for myself but for LeBron as well so that I can maximize our nutritional options.

- First, I'll check what the hotel offers for breakfast. If it consists of nothing but pastries and bagels, I'll find a supermarket within walking distance (or one that delivers for a small fee), as well as a couple healthy eateries and restaurants.
- Next, I'll call the hotel and ask if there is a refrigerator in my room and what its size is. If there isn't, I'll ask for one (even if it means switching rooms) so I have more storage options for healthy foods I'll find when I'm there. You'd be surprised how easy it is for most hotels to accommodate that.
- After that, I'll get a lay of the land to find out what restaurants may be potential places to eat based on location, then look at menus ahead of time to verify which offer the widest assortment of healthy choices.
- Finally, I'll do some research about certain events that take place only on certain days—such as farmer's markets or festivals—that may provide a few other nutritious, fresher options I may want to stock up on and have at hand during my stay.

The point is, in my experience of traveling for decades to countless cities around the world for my job, I can safely say that better nutritional choices are always around you, no matter where you are. It's really a matter of figuring out what options are available to you *before* you get to your destination.

You're likely traveling for work, pleasure, or some other event that's fighting for your time and attention. By arriving prepared, you'll never put yourself in the position of feeling like you're rushing to decide, wasting time you may not have, or holding anybody up. Because it's during those moments that you can make poorer decisions you'll regret once you're back home. You need to feel confident that wherever you are, you can quickly and conveniently pull off what you know is best for your body nutritionally. Because if you don't, you'll pull yourself back performance-wise instead of being ahead of the game.

If all this sounds like a lot of work, it can be—that's what preparation is! That's why I like to keep it simple for my clients by having them follow what I call **"figure out your future meal."** Meaning, after every single meal or snack, before you throw your dish in the sink or pull the napkin off your lap, ask yourself, *"Where exactly will I be two to three hours from now?"* Because wherever that place is—that's the place that ultimately decides whether it's going to be easier or harder for you to eat healthier when hunger strikes. In that moment, consider the following:

- Is there anything you can foresee that might prevent you from making the best nutritional choices in a few hours, and if so, can you plan right now to prevent that from happening?
- Will you be someplace where eating might be impossible or inconvenient, and if that's the case, can you pack something now, so you have more healthier options at your fingertips?

Instead of just going from point A to point B—even if that journey doesn't have you moving an inch from your desk chair or your living room couch—spend a few minutes before you leave point A to consider what will be available to you along that journey *before* you take it.

Amplify those around you. If having lunch with someone who eats healthy is what has helped keep you on track, I entirely get it. Imagine what it's like for me being around LeBron and the other players on the team, finding myself always in the company of some of the world's greatest athletes, as well as many of the top experts in human performance, dietetics, strength and conditioning, and so forth. I'll tell you this—it makes it hard to reach for a bag of chips without feeling a little self-conscious. And it makes it a little bit easier to grab an apple and a handful of almonds, surrounded as I am by athletes that are a testament to the power of clean, nutritious eating.

As I mentioned in the last chapter, if you have people in your life who eat healthy and inspire you to do the same when around them, then be around them as often as possible. But if that's easier said than done, you can still use those rocks in other ways, even when they're not sitting across from you:

- **Tell your meal to smile for the camera.** Strike a deal with a few of your rocks to send them a picture of any meal or snack before you eat it. You can make it a daily thing or just on certain days or meals that may be more difficult for you to stay the course. Either way, doing so brings accountability to that meal *in* the moment, making you less likely to make poor choices and more likely to make smart ones to impress. In fact, consider competing against your rocks to see who can eat the healthiest meal that day.
- **Ask yourself, "What would [insert friend's name here] eat?"** If you don't have access to your rocks for some reason, pause for a moment and consider what they might choose at that period. Take it a step further and imagine you're buying that meal for them so that the pressure's on.
- **Confess your nutritional sins.** So many people might acknowledge their mistakes after eating a bad meal to themselves but are less likely to admit it to others. That's because sometimes guilt turns into shame that keeps them from wanting to admit they messed up. Or they don't want to appear weaker in the eyes of those around them. All I know is, that shouldn't be you. If you screwed up a meal (and you know why after breaking it down), I want you to immediately reach out to a few of your rocks and share that information. Here's why:

- ◦ The more you talk to your friends about how you tripped up with your diet, the stronger your understanding will become of that mistake—and the less likely you'll be to make it again.
- ◦ Your rocks may know of other ways you could avoid repeating that same mistake that you're not thinking about.

Amplify your curiosity. I have a saying: "If you're 'bored' with your options, then you haven't 'explored' your options." It applies to many things in life but particularly diet. For example, when I hear people say they hate vegetables, I explain how that's statistically impossible because there's simply no way any human being could hate 20,000 things, particularly 20,000 things they've most likely never tried.

You read that right. That's how many edible vegetables are out there to choose from, a number that stuns a lot of people who couldn't list even a few dozen veggies if I asked them to. The same goes for fruit. Like berries? There are more than 400 kinds you could choose from. What about apples? At last count, you're looking at 7,500 varieties to choose from. Pick any common fruit such as bananas (1,000 and counting), cherries (roughly 1,200), and even grapes (10,000+), and you could spend a lifetime attempting to try every variety.

Now, it's true: Your local grocery store probably doesn't stock 10,000 different types of grapes. But that doesn't mean you can't put a little elbow grease into expanding your palette:

- **Ask for what's in season or nonlocal.** Whether it's at a supermarket, a farmer's market, or a restaurant, inquiring about either will point you in the direction of foods typically not as common for you to experience.
- **Find every ethnic grocery store in your area.** Latin, Mexican, Middle Eastern, Indian, Pan-Asian, Serbian, Jamaican, and so on—all of them will carry meats, vegetables, fruits, nuts, and seeds that you're unlikely to find at a conventional supermarket. Visit a different one every week and don't be afraid to ask the owners for suggestions.

Amplify your atmosphere. If the ambience you chose the last time you ate helped put you in the mood for the right kind of food, stick with it. If it wasn't, there are a few ways you can give yourself an atmospheric edge when it comes to your eating.

- **Turn up the lights.** Forsaking a candlelit meal for one illuminated by fluorescent bulbs may not be as romantic, but it can be the right choice to keep the wrong things from finding their way onto your plate. Most people tend to eat more in dim or dark places, not just because they're less self-conscious about what's in front of them—I mean, if you can barely see your food, how can the person at the next table?—but because lower lighting can leave us feeling more relaxed, which tends to drop inhibitions just a bit when it comes to eating.
- **Look for the three B's.** It turns out that brown, black, and dark blue have a secret superpower: They suppress appetite. (On the other hand, brighter colors, such as red, orange, yellow, and green, have the opposite effect.) I'm not saying break out the paint cans in your kitchen, but at the very least, consider where you're seated (and what you're facing) when at home or dining out to give yourself even more of an atmospheric leg up.

Dial Back Your Defeats

So maybe the situation got out of your control—who cares? It's not your first time and it definitely won't be your last. The good news is you've broken down how your ship went off course, which automatically will make it less likely to happen the next time. Still, rethinking whatever obstacles knocked you backward can help improve your chances of moving forward the next time. Even though the last chapter offered some solutions to think about as you broke down what went wrong, there are some additional considerations you could make with a few particular obstacles.

Dial back your lack of time. In the last chapter, I gave you a couple things to consider, including looking for the wasted minutes in your day and retracing your steps. But are there other tricks to try? Honestly, I know plenty, and I'm sure you do too, because most of them revolve around food preparation I'm sure you've heard about before. Deciding beforehand what you're going to eat during the next few days, loading up your house with what you need, cooking foods ahead of time, filling your freezer with vegetables and fruits already washed, peeled, and cut—all the obvious ways to have healthier choices at the ready. But there are a few hacks that people don't seem to talk about much:

- **Buy a decent-sized cooler.** Most of the time, what we reach for when we're in a rush are convenient foods. But what makes them convenient has less to do with their proximity and more to do with the preservatives inside them and processes they undergo that keep them from rotting, just so we can keep them in our desk drawers when needed. Instead, I want you to make healthy choices more convenient by investing in an insulated cooler. Not the type that barely holds a sandwich and a small water bottle, but one big enough that allows you to keep healthy fare in your car, office, or wherever you find yourself needing to eat healthier, especially if healthy options aren't close by.
- **Grab your take-out menus and circle the good stuff.** In most cases, if you're reaching for one, it's usually because you don't have time to prepare a meal. So, doesn't it make sense in that kind of high-pressure situation to know ahead of time the best choices that match your longevity goals? By circling the smartest options on every menu you might reach for at a later date, you're guaranteeing your chances of ordering what your body needs in a pinch versus letting lack of time cause a nutritional choice you might later regret. The same rule applies if you prefer to pull menus up on your phone rather than out of a kitchen drawer. If that's you, then simply scroll through the menus of places

you already frequent (or most likely will in the future), find the healthiest option, and screenshot it so you have it among your photos to refer to when needed.

- **Become a portion-size pro.** A lot of my clients don't like to count grams or ounces—and who can blame them? But that makes it more difficult to determine whether you're eating an actual serving of lean protein, complex carbohydrates, or healthy fats. That's why I have them compare portion sizes against objects they already know. For example:
  - An average serving (3 ounces) of cooked chicken, fish, or meat? Easy—picture the size of a woman's palm or a deck of cards.
  - An average serving of nuts or seeds (1 ounce) is roughly what you can put in your hand. Mind you, I'm talking about an average guy's hand—not the size of most NBA players I know—so if you've got some big mitts of your own, try pouring in an ounce of nuts or seeds into your palm so you can see how much real estate it takes up.
  - For an average serving of cooked rice or pasta (1 cup) or a single serving of fruit or vegetables, skip the measuring cup and imagine the size of a tennis ball.
  - To measure an average serving of oil (1 teaspoon), give yourself a big thumbs-up! The end of your thumb—from the tip to the first knuckle—is pretty much the same size.
  - Don't see any comparisons for other healthy foods you've been eating regularly? Then take the time when you have a few minutes to measure out one serving of whatever it is, then make a mental note of what the size looks like. That way the next time you're in a rush and need to put together a meal, you can forget the measuring cups and scales and just go by eyeballing it.
- **Finally, ask yourself—what am I really saving in the long run?** Maybe visiting that drive-thru gave you ten minutes you thought you didn't have or grabbing that doughnut with your coffee kept you from having to waste fifteen minutes making a decent

healthy breakfast. But whenever I hear a client say things like that, I remind them that whenever you *think* you're saving time, if that time comes at the expense of your own health, then you'll have to make it up later.

What do I mean by that? I want you to consider that drive-thru run or that doughnut—or whatever poor food choice you made because you were rushed or impatient—and really boil down exactly how many minutes you saved. Then ask yourself:

- Will you need to exercise or be active for at least that long to burn off whatever came with that choice? If extending your longevity truly is your goal, the unhealthy fats, chemicals, and extra calories typically within these foods just means you'll be spending even more time than you saved working it off through exercise and watching your diet later.
- Were you less efficient later that day because you felt more sluggish and tired as a result of not fueling yourself the right way? That means your initial effort to be more productive by sparing yourself time only came back to sabotage your progress in a different area in your life.
- Did you potentially shorten your own life span by a few minutes—just because you couldn't wait or spend a few extra minutes? This is a question that's impossible to answer right away because the cumulative effects of eating poorly take time. But both science and common sense would point to yes.

Dial back your tension. The good news is, by incorporating my mobility program into your life and being more proactive about how your body heals, you'll naturally reduce your stress levels and be less likely to reach for comfort foods and other unhealthy choices. However, neither is the perfect solution for relieving whatever might be causing you to stress eat—and only you can uncover that cause. That's why identifying those sources of tension as quickly as possible—and figuring out a way to either reduce or remove them from your life—is so important.

- **Find the cause and bring it closure.** Now, if you're going through something that's not easy to quickly address, that's entirely understandable. But if there's anything that's within your control to change or put an end to, that's what you need to target and take care of:
    - If it's something you're putting off, then immediately make it your top priority.
    - If it's something you can't get around to right away, then identify when you will have time and mark it on your calendar so you feel that you have a handle on it at the very least.

Make the Mix Even Better!

If you commit to eating five to six meals or snacks daily—each made up of one serving of lean protein, one serving of complex carbohydrates, and one serving of healthy fats—you'll be lightyears ahead of your competition. You'll be matching the diets of most elite athletes. But is there a way to squeeze out a little more benefit from this three-part mix? There is—it just depends on what type of day you're going to have tomorrow.

Low-Energy Versus High-Energy Days

Typical lifestyle programs (or dare I say the word *diets*) suggest the same "five days on/two days off" food schedule. You know what I'm talking about. You might be told to eat a particular way Monday through Friday, but on weekends, the rules change, and you're allowed a little more slack to account for life getting in the way.

But that's not life at all. When you look at that type of agenda, you're being asked to eat a stricter diet on weekdays, days when you may need more energy to get you through. Meanwhile, you're allowed to eat more on weekends, two days where you may be a little less active—and require fewer calories—because you're relaxing from a long work week. On the other hand, your work/life schedule could be just like mine and my clients: working on certain days when most people are off (and vice versa), stepping onto the court when most people are stepping into their pj's, or busy on the road 24/7 for months on end before catching a breather.

What I know is this: Everyone's nutritional demands are their own, and they can change in an instant depending on what the week throws at you. That's why you can't just arbitrarily break down your diet into weekdays versus weekends. Instead, it's smarter to categorize your week by looking forward and asking yourself if tomorrow is going to be a "high-performance" day or a "low-/average-performance" day. In other words, you need to think ahead and recognize whether:

- Your body will require a little more energy tomorrow (which you could prepare for today by eating a little more carbohydrates—and fully topping off your glycogen stores).
- Or, since your body may not require as much energy tomorrow, it could benefit from eating a little cleaner today and focusing more on lean protein to rebuild itself back up even better than before.

For example, maybe Monday, Tuesday, Thursday, and Saturday, you don't have much going on. But Wednesday, Friday, and Sunday, well, those are the three busiest days of your week. Maybe Wednesday, you have a big presentation where you'll need to be as alert as possible to stand up in front of people for an hour. And Friday, that's the day you planned on blowing off steam after work by playing a doubleheader in your softball league. And then there's Sunday, the day you're finally getting around to cleaning out your garage.

See my point? Every week is different, and to have that weekday/weekend divide with your diet is a quick way to ensure you might not have enough energy on certain days when you really need it, as well as lack enough nutrients to heal on other days when your body requires more nutrients. Even if you're not an athlete, thinking like an athlete—putting a little thought into what your body might need the next day, and then tweaking the mixture of macronutrients (protein, complex carbs, and healthy fats) the day before so that those nutrients are in your system and ready to go—is all it takes.

Ideally, to give yourself enough time to prepare certain meals or foods, you could look ahead to sort of gauge how active you expect to be over the next three days or so. But since my clients oftentimes get surprised by situations where they may need to take on unexpected events, activities, or meetings, I like to teach people to think even more in the short term and focus on tomorrow.

Instead of waking up and wondering what you'll eat *that day*, I want you getting in the practice of eating with an eye toward whatever *tomorrow* is going to be like for you. In other words, recognizing if you'll need more energy to take on tomorrow (because it's going to be a busier day than usual) or if you'll need more nutrients to help your body heal faster by taking advantage of a typical or more relaxed day.

If all of this sounds complex, it's not—or I should say it doesn't have to be. Here is the simplified version I recommend to clients:

If tomorrow is a *high*-performance day for you . . .

. . . then what I want you to do *today* is carbo-fortify—in other words, eat a little more complex carbohydrates than recommended in Chapter 4—to make sure both your brain and body have more energy than usual the next day.

What do I consider to be a high-performance day? It's basically a day with an event that you believe will require a significant amount of energy, whether physically or mentally, for at least ninety minutes or more.

Now, I know what you're going to say: "Mike, that's every day for me." Of course, we all feel that way sometimes. And sure, there are certain weeks that we run ourselves into the ground 24/7. But when you honestly step back and look at the next few days ahead of you, it doesn't take much to spot which ones might be a little more intense than others. There are days when you need to be at your absolute best when it comes to your energy because it could have a negative impact on your life if you're not. Those are the ones I would consider high-performance days.

So what should you eat the day before a high-performance day? You may already be familiar with the expression *carbo-loading*, a tactic that many athletes use before endurance events—particularly ones lasting longer than ninety minutes such as half-marathons, marathons, long-distance bike races, etc. It's basically a process where athletes taper back and/or step away from activity/exercise while consuming more carbohydrates than normal over the course of three to six days. What's the point? To build up the stored glycogen in their bodies above its normal capacity so that they have a little more energy to tap in to on race day.

That—by the way—is *not* what I'm going to have you do. Instead, what you can try (if you're curious to) is just a slight modification to your meals and snacks the day before a high-performance day by taking in more carbohydrates than usual—just to make sure your glycogen stores are tapped off.

So instead of having one of the following at every meal or snack:

- One serving of high-quality protein
- One serving of complex carbohydrates
- One serving of healthy fats

. . . you're going to eat as usual all day long until dinner, and that's when you'll switch the mix to:

- One serving of high-quality protein
- Two servings of complex carbohydrates (ideally from grains or higher-caloric fruits and vegetables)
- One serving of healthy fats

If tomorrow is a *low*-performance day for you . . .

. . . then what I want you to do *today* is limit high-density carbohydrates and load up on more lean protein to fortify your body with even more of what it needs to rebuild itself.

What do I consider a "low-performance" day? I would say it's one where you don't expect any big surprises to come your way that require much physical exertion or serious brain power—a day when you know you'll be relaxed more than revved up.

The day before a low-performance day, you'll eat as usual all day long until dinner, and then switch things around in the following way:

- Two servings of high-quality protein
- One serving of complex carbohydrates (strictly from low-caloric vegetables)
- One to two servings of healthy fats

If you have no idea what kind of day tomorrow will be . . .

. . . then what I want you to do *today* is stick with the original game plan and eat the following at every meal or snack . . .

- One serving of high-quality protein
- One serving of complex carbohydrates (your choice)
- One serving of healthy fats

Last Points

Is this an exact science? No! And, in fact, I fully expect some nutritionists to discount this solution of preparing yourself for the next day. But I defy you to find one method of eating that all nutritionists agree with—because everybody takes a different approach to eating.

Will you always feel a huge difference? Sometimes you will, but some days the effects might only be slight. But each extra little bit helps.

Finally, do you have to try it? Absolutely not, especially if you feel it will only make your day more challenging or confusing. The regular method will give you a decent enough approximation. But most clients find this tweak helpful if they give it a shot. Just know that if you decide to stick with the original formula and not factor in high- versus low-performance days, you're still eating a mix of macronutrients that, left on their own, are already putting you well ahead of the curve, thanks to the abundance of vitamins, minerals, fiber, and crucial nutrients that support performance, health, and longevity.

Menus

To make it even easier for you to fuel up without having to think too much about it, I asked Chef Mary Shenouda—one of the most-sought-after performance chefs and nutritional consultants in the business—for some unique recipes that capture my low-/high-performance day philosophy.

Chef Mary has worked with and continues to advise some of the biggest names in sports and entertainment, including athletes on the Golden State Warriors (contributing to their 2022 NBA Championship), pro soccer player Javier "Chicharito" Hernández, Academy Award–winner Lupita Nyong'o, WWE superstar Mike "The Miz" Mizanin, and many other A-list celebrities through EPC Performance, her consultancy.

Mary is also the creator and founder of Phat Fudge (her performance nutrition line) and the host of the *Eat Play Crush* podcast, which is focused on making wellness and performance relatable through interviews with experts. In addition, Chef Mary is also a product formulator for the nationally distributed brands Primal Kitchen and Safe Harvest, a contributor to several bestselling books (including *The Genius Life*, *Genius Kitchen*, and *How to Conceive Naturally: And Have a Healthy Pregnancy After 30*), as well as a consultant for brands such as Nike, Oura Health, and Hyperice.

Working with a team of doctors, physical therapists, specialty-focused practitioners, nutritionists, and performance technologies, Chef Mary is as passionate as I am about helping individuals reach their full potential and believes that nutrition is the foundational pillar in achieving success. Her ability to identify and curate the specific nutritional and recovery needs of her clients on a micronutrient level—then create delicious meals that help them perform at their peak—is why she was my top choice for constructing the best possible recipes for this book.

A Note from Chef Mary Shenouda

When Mike asked me to contribute to his book, it was an easy yes. Aside from his being a rock-solid human being, there are very few professionals as committed to their craft while also being generous with their time and expertise as Mike—and that's why I'm thrilled to share these recipes with you. Use them as a guide for other potential ways to incorporate his diet philosophy into your life while having fun in the kitchen so you can eat well, play hard, and crush your life. Trust your gut!

Overnight Chia Pudding (sweet)

MAKES 1 SERVING

Calories: 200–300
Protein: 10–15 grams
Carbohydrates: 30–35 grams
Fat: 10–15 grams

This breakfast consists of just a few simple ingredients and can be prepped ahead of time, so it's a perfect grab-and-go option. Chia seeds are a great source of protein, fiber, and omega-3 fatty acids, making them a nutrient-rich way to start your day.

Ingredients

3 tablespoons chia seeds

1 cup unsweetened almond milk (or any nondairy milk)

1 tablespoon honey or maple syrup, plus more to taste

1/4 teaspoon vanilla extract

Fresh fruit and nuts, for serving

Instructions

1. In a small bowl or jar, combine the chia seeds, almond milk, honey or maple syrup, and vanilla extract. Mix well.
2. Cover the bowl or jar and refrigerate overnight or for at least 4 hours, until the chia seeds have absorbed the liquid and formed a pudding-like consistency.
3. Stir the chia pudding before serving and adjust the sweetness, if desired. Top with fresh fruit and nuts of your choice.
4. Enjoy chilled.

Gluten-Free Banana Pancakes (sweet)

MAKES 2 PANCAKES (1 SERVING)

Calories: 300–330
Protein: 10–15 grams
Carbohydrates: 40–45 grams
Fat: 10–15 grams

These gluten-free banana pancakes are a great way to start your day. They're packed with protein and carbohydrates, which will give you the energy you need to power through your day.

The bananas in these pancakes are a good source of potassium, which is an important mineral for muscle function. The eggs also provide protein, which is essential for repairing and building muscle tissue. And the oat flour is a good source of fiber, which will help you feel full and satisfied.

Ingredients

1 ripe banana, mashed
2 eggs
1/4 cup gluten-free oat flour
1/4 teaspoon baking powder
1/4 teaspoon vanilla extract
Pinch of salt
Cooking spray or oil, for greasing the pan
Fresh berries and a drizzle of honey, for serving

Instructions

1. In a mixing bowl, combine the mashed banana, eggs, oat flour, baking powder, vanilla extract, and salt. Stir until well combined.
2. Heat a small nonstick skillet or griddle over medium heat and lightly grease it with cooking spray or oil.
3. Spoon about 1/2 cup of the pancake batter onto the pan. Cook for 2 to 3 minutes, until bubbles form on the surface, then flip and cook for another 1 to 2 minutes, until golden brown.
4. Repeat with the remaining batter.
5. Serve the pancakes with fresh berries and a drizzle of honey.

Green Smoothie Bowl (sweet)

MAKES 1 SERVING

Calories: 300–350
Protein: 10–15 grams
Carbohydrates: 40–45 grams
Fat: 10–15 grams

This green smoothie bowl is packed with nutrients that will fuel your body for a day of activity. The frozen banana provides natural sweetness and creaminess, while the spinach or kale leaves add a boost of vitamins, minerals, and antioxidants. The almond milk, almond butter, and chia seeds also provide protein and healthy fats to keep you feeling full and satisfied.

Ingredients

1 frozen banana

1 cup spinach or kale leaves

1/2 cup unsweetened almond milk or any other nondairy milk, plus more as needed

1 tablespoon almond butter or peanut butter

1 tablespoon chia seeds

Sliced fresh fruit, shredded coconut, granola, and/or nuts, for topping

Instructions

1. In a blender, combine the frozen banana, spinach or kale leaves, almond milk, almond butter or peanut butter, and chia seeds. Blend until smooth and creamy. Add more almond milk if needed to reach the desired consistency.
2. Pour the smoothie into a bowl. Top with sliced fresh fruit, shredded coconut, granola, and/or nuts.
3. Enjoy with a spoon.

Sweet Potato and Veggie (Mostly) Egg White Scramble (savory)

MAKES 1 SERVING

Calories: 450–480
Protein: 36 grams
Carbohydrates: 50–60 grams
Fat: 20–25 grams

This bowl is packed with protein, carbohydrates, and healthy fats. It's a great way to start your day before a workout. The sweet potatoes are a good source of fiber and beta-carotene, an antioxidant that can help protect your cells from damage. The other vegetables add even more nutrients, and the egg whites provide protein without a lot of fat, while including one egg yolk helps with overall digestion.

Ingredients

1 large (8 ounces) sweet potato, peeled and diced into 1/2-inch pieces
1/4 cup chopped red bell pepper
1/4 cup chopped spinach
1/4 cup sliced mushrooms
1/4 cup diced tomatoes
3 egg whites
1 whole egg
Salt and pepper to taste
1 tablespoon extra-virgin olive oil
Fresh fruit, for serving

Instructions

1. Over medium heat, sauté the sweet potatoes in olive oil, covered, for 2 to 3 minutes.
2. Add the bell pepper, spinach, mushrooms, and tomatoes to the pan. Sauté for 2 to 3 minutes until the vegetables soften.
3. In a medium bowl, whisk the egg whites and whole egg until frothy. Season with salt and pepper.
4. Pour the eggs over the sautéed vegetables in the pan. Allow it to cook for 2 to 3 minutes, until the edges are set.
5. Gently fold the omelet in half and cook for another minute until it's fully cooked.
6. Serve hot with a side of fresh fruit.

Berry Quinoa Breakfast Bowl (sweet)

MAKES 1 SERVING

Calories: 400–450
Protein: 15–20 grams
Carbohydrates: 60–70 grams
Fat: 10–15 grams

This quinoa breakfast bowl is packed with protein, fiber, and complex carbohydrates to keep you feeling full and energized all morning long. It's also a great source of antioxidants and vitamins, thanks to the mixed berries and chia seeds.

Ingredients

1/2 cup cooked quinoa

1/4 cup unsweetened almond milk

1 tablespoon honey or maple syrup

1/4 cup mixed berries (such as blueberries, strawberries, and raspberries)

1 tablespoon chia seeds

1 tablespoon sliced almonds

1 teaspoon ground cinnamon (optional)

Instructions

1. In a small saucepan over low heat, warm the cooked quinoa and almond milk for a minute or two. Stir in the honey or maple syrup until well combined.
2. Transfer the quinoa mixture to a serving bowl. Top with the mixed berries, chia seeds, and sliced almonds. Sprinkle with cinnamon, if desired.
3. Enjoy warm or chilled.

Greek Yogurt Parfait (sweet)

MAKES 1 SERVING

Calories: 300–350
Protein: 20–25 grams
Carbohydrates: 30–35 grams
Fat: 10–15 grams

This recipe is a great source of protein, which will help you feel full and satisfied throughout the morning. The fruit provides essential vitamins and minerals, and the granola adds fiber and healthy fats.

Ingredients

1 cup plain Greek yogurt or dairy-free yogurt

1/2 cup mixed fresh fruit (such as berries, sliced banana, and diced mango)

2 tablespoons gluten-free granola

1 tablespoon honey or maple syrup

1 tablespoon unsweetened coconut flakes (optional)

Instructions

1. In a glass or small bowl, spread half of the Greek yogurt on the bottom. Add half of the mixed fresh fruit on top of the yogurt.
2. Sprinkle 1 tablespoon of the granola over the fruit. Drizzle 1/2 tablespoon of the honey on top.
3. Repeat the layers with the remaining ingredients. Top with unsweetened coconut flakes, if desired.
4. Enjoy immediately.

Spicy Shrimp Lettuce Wraps

MAKES 4 WRAPS (1 SERVING)

Calories: 280
Protein: 25 grams
Carbohydrates: 8 grams
Fat: 15 grams

These spicy shrimp lettuce wraps are a zesty and refreshing option for a low-carb, high-protein lunch. The succulent shrimp are seasoned with a tantalizing blend of spices, including cayenne pepper for a kick. Wrapped in crisp lettuce leaves, these wraps are not only gluten-free but also low in calories. It's a satisfying meal that won't weigh you down, perfect for a low-activity day when you're looking for a lighter lunch option.

Ingredients

1 teaspoon extra-virgin olive oil

1/2 teaspoon paprika

1/4 teaspoon cayenne pepper

1/4 teaspoon garlic powder

Salt and pepper to taste

8 large shrimp, peeled and deveined

4 large lettuce leaves, such as butter lettuce or romaine

1/4 cup diced tomatoes

1/4 cup diced red onions

2 tablespoons chopped fresh cilantro

1 tablespoon fresh lime juice

Hot sauce or sriracha, for extra spice (optional)

Instructions

1. In a bowl, combine the olive oil, paprika, cayenne pepper, garlic powder, and salt and pepper. Toss the shrimp in the spice mixture until coated evenly.
2. Heat a nonstick skillet over medium heat. Add the shrimp and cook for 2 to 3 minutes on each side until pink and opaque.
3. Once cooked, remove the shrimp from the skillet and let them cool slightly.
4. Take a lettuce leaf and place a few shrimp in the center. Top with diced tomatoes, red onions, cilantro, and a drizzle of lime juice.
5. Repeat with the remaining lettuce leaves and shrimp. For some extra heat, add a few dashes of hot sauce or sriracha.
6. Roll up the lettuce leaves and enjoy these flavorful and protein-packed spicy shrimp wraps!

Greek Chicken Salad

MAKES 1 SERVING

Calories: 350
Protein: 30 grams
Carbohydrates: 10 grams
Fat: 20 grams

Packed with fresh ingredients and loaded with protein, this is a satisfying and healthy lunch option. The tender grilled chicken is combined with crisp cucumbers, juicy tomatoes, tangy feta cheese, and a homemade Greek dressing. This gluten-free and low-carb salad is perfect for a low-activity day when you're aiming for a lighter meal without sacrificing flavor.

Ingredients

2 cups mixed salad greens

1 small grilled skinless, boneless chicken breast (4 ounces), sliced

1/2 cucumber, sliced

1/2 cup cherry tomatoes, halved

1/4 cup crumbled feta cheese or dairy-free alternative

2 tablespoons kalamata olives, pitted and sliced

2 tablespoons chopped red onion

2 tablespoons chopped fresh parsley

Greek Dressing

2 tablespoons extra-virgin olive oil

1 tablespoon fresh lemon juice

1 teaspoon red wine vinegar

1/2 teaspoon dried oregano

Salt and pepper to taste

Instructions

1. In a large bowl, combine the mixed salad greens, sliced grilled chicken, cucumber slices, cherry tomatoes, crumbled feta cheese, kalamata olives, chopped red onion, and fresh parsley.
2. In a small bowl, whisk together the olive oil, lemon juice, red wine vinegar, dried oregano, and salt and pepper.
3. Drizzle the dressing over the salad and toss gently to coat all the ingredients.
4. Serve right away!

Zucchini Noodle Stir-Fry with Tempeh

MAKES 1 SERVING

Calories: 300
Protein: 25 grams
Carbohydrates: 15 grams
Fat: 18 grams

By replacing traditional noodles with zucchini noodles, or "zoodles," you can enjoy a flavorful, gluten-free, and low-carb lunch that's packed with protein. The tempeh adds a hearty and plant-based protein source, while the colorful array of veggies provides essential nutrients. This dish is perfect for a low activity day when you want a lighter meal without compromising taste or satiety.

Ingredients

1 tablespoon sesame oil
6 ounces tempeh, cubed
2 garlic cloves, minced
1 red bell pepper, sliced
1 carrot, julienned
1/2 cup snow peas
2 green onions, sliced
2 tablespoons gluten-free soy sauce or tamari
1 tablespoon rice vinegar
1/2 teaspoon grated fresh ginger
1/4 teaspoon red pepper flakes (optional)
1 large zucchini, spiralized into noodles
1 tablespoon sesame seeds, for garnish

Instructions

1. In a large skillet or wok, heat the sesame oil over medium heat. Add the cubed tempeh and cook until golden brown on all sides. Remove the tempeh from the skillet and set aside.
2. In the same skillet, add the garlic, red bell pepper, carrot, snow peas, and green onions. Stir-fry for 2 to 3 minutes, until the vegetables are slightly tender.
3. In a small bowl, whisk together the gluten-free soy sauce or tamari, rice vinegar, grated ginger, and the red pepper flakes, if desired. Pour the sauce over the stir-fried vegetables and toss to coat.
4. Add the zucchini noodles and cooked tempeh to the skillet. Gently toss everything together and cook for an additional 2 minutes, until the zucchini noodles are tender but still have a slight crunch.
5. Remove from the heat and sprinkle with the sesame seeds for added texture and flavor.
6. Serve the zucchini noodle stir-fry while it's still warm.

Chicken and Avocado Quinoa Power Bowl

MAKES 1 SERVING

Calories: 600
Protein: 34 grams
Carbohydrates: 43 grams
Fat: 50 grams

This gluten-free delight is packed with complex carbs and moderate protein to fuel your high-activity day. Start with a fluffy bed of quinoa, and pile on the grilled chicken thighs, roasted sweet potatoes, and steamed broccoli. Top it off with creamy avocado slices and a sprinkle of chopped almonds for added crunch. Drizzle the lemon vinaigrette over the bowl, giving it a tangy kick that will make your taste buds dance.

Ingredients

1 cup quinoa, cooked in broth

2 grilled boneless, skinless chicken thighs (5 ounces), diced

1 cup roasted sweet potato cubes

1 cup steamed broccoli florets

1/4 cup sliced avocado

2 tablespoons chopped almonds

1 tablespoon lemon juice

1 tablespoon extra-virgin olive oil

Salt and pepper to taste

Instructions

Toss all the ingredients together and enjoy.

Lemon-Poached Halibut with Roasted Potatoes

MAKES 1 SERVING

Calories: 500
Protein: 23 grams
Carbohydrates: 80 grams
Fat: 15 grams

This recipe is simple, yet has sophisticated flavors. Imagine: tender halibut, infused with the essence of lemon and oregano, nestled amid a bed of crispy roasted fingerling potatoes. Tangy tomatoes burst with sweetness, while pops of salty capers add their flavor. It's a perfect balance of textures and tastes, all coming together in a single pan for easy cleanup.

Ingredients

2 pounds fingerling potatoes, halved

Extra-virgin olive oil

Salt and pepper

6 ounces halibut fillet

1/4 teaspoon dried oregano

1 lemon, sliced

16 ounces grape tomatoes, half a portion of them

1 tablespoon minced fresh parsley

1 tablespoon capers

Instructions

1. Place the rack in the middle of the oven, and preheat the oven to 450°F.
2. In a medium bowl, toss the potatoes with 2 tablespoons olive oil, 1/2 teaspoon salt, and 1/4 teaspoon pepper.
3. On a baking sheet, arrange the potatoes cut side down and roast until slightly brown, 15 to 22 minutes.
4. Meanwhile, make a foil packet and place the halibut inside (do a search online to see how), and then add some olive oil, the oregano, a pinch of salt, a slice of lemon, and the tomatoes.
5. Remove the baking sheet from the oven and place the halibut packet on top of the potatoes, returning the baking sheet to the oven for another 10 to 15 minutes.
6. Remove the baking sheet from the oven again. Open the foil packet carefully to make sure the steam releases away from you. Slide the halibut out of the packet, then pour the rest of the juices and tomatoes over the potatoes.
7. Serve everything together with additional fresh lemon slices and the parsley and capers.

Red Lentil Lettuce Cups

MAKES 1 SERVING

Calories: 460
Protein: 18 grams
Carbohydrates: 62 grams
Fat: 18 grams

The hearty lentils, infused with warm spices and a touch of lemon zest, offer a satisfying bite, while the fresh vegetables and creamy yogurt provide a delightful contrast in texture and flavor—these red lentil lettuce cups will hit the spot and your macros.

Ingredients

1/4 cup extra-virgin olive oil
1 sweet onion, minced
1/2 red bell pepper, finely chopped
1/2 teaspoon sea salt, plus more to taste
1 tablespoon harissa
1 tablespoon tomato paste
1/2 cup fonio or quinoa
2 cups bone broth
1/2 cup dried red lentils, rinsed
1 tablespoon fresh lemon juice
1/4 cup chopped fresh parsley
Black pepper to taste
1/2 head of Bibb lettuce
2/3 cup plain yogurt or dairy-free yogurt, for serving
Lemon wedges, for serving

Instructions

1. In a large saucepan, heat the olive oil over medium heat. Sauté the onions, bell pepper, and salt until the vegetables are lightly golden brown.
2. Add the harissa and tomato paste, stirring until well combined.
3. Stir in the fonio or quinoa and the bone broth and bring to a boil. Reduce the heat and let cook until the grains are tender.
4. Stir in the lentils, cover, and cook for 8 to 10 minutes, stirring occasionally, until the lentils are tender.
5. Remove the pan from the heat and let everything rest for 10 minutes.
6. Add the lemon juice and parsley, and season with salt and black pepper.
7. To serve, scoop the lentil mixture into lettuce cups and serve with yogurt and lemon wedges.

Gluten-Free Turkey Meatballs with Spaghetti Squash

MAKES 4 SERVINGS

Calories: 420
Protein: 30 grams
Carbohydrates: 34 grams
Fat: 16 grams

This recipe is a healthier twist on the classic spaghetti-and-meatballs dish. The turkey meatballs are made with gluten-free breadcrumbs and are baked instead of fried, while the spaghetti squash is a great low-carb alternative to traditional pasta. This recipe is also a good source of protein and fiber, and a relatively low-fat option.

Ingredients

1 pound ground turkey

1/2 cup gluten-free breadcrumbs

1 egg, beaten

1/4 cup grated Parmesan cheese or dairy-free alternative

1 teaspoon Italian seasoning

1/2 teaspoon salt

1/4 teaspoon pepper

1/2 cup marinara sauce

1 medium spaghetti squash, baked and forked out (do an online search to see how)

Instructions

1. Preheat the oven to 400°F.
2. In a large bowl, combine the ground turkey, breadcrumbs, egg, Parmesan cheese, Italian seasoning, salt, and pepper. Mix until well combined.
3. With wet hands, form the turkey mixture into 1-inch meatballs and place on a baking sheet. Bake for 18 to 20 minutes.
4. Toss the meatballs with the marinara sauce and serve with spaghetti squash.

Savory Beef and Macaroni

MAKES 1 SERVING

Calories: 530
Protein: 35 grams
Carbohydrates: 66 grams
Fat: 16 grams

This savory beef and macaroni is a hearty and flavorful dish that's perfect for a quick and easy weeknight meal. It's packed with protein and fiber, and it's low in carbohydrates. This recipe is also gluten-free, so it's perfect for people with dietary restrictions.

Ingredients

1/2 sweet onion, chopped

2 tablespoons extra-virgin olive oil

1 tomato, diced

1 garlic clove, minced

1 teaspoon finely ground espresso

1 tablespoon chili powder, plus more to taste

1 teaspoon garlic powder, plus more to taste

1/2 teaspoon ground cloves, plus more to taste

1 teaspoon salt, plus more to taste

6 ounces ground beef

2 tablespoons tomato paste

1 tablespoon coconut aminos or or soy sauce (preferably tamari, a gluten-free version)

1/2 lemon

1 cup gluten-free elbow macaroni, cooked

Instructions

1. In a large pot, brown the onions in the olive oil over medium heat.
2. Add the diced tomatoes and cook until soft.
3. Mix in the minced garlic, espresso, chili powder, garlic powder, cloves, and salt, and cook until fragrant.
4. Add the ground beef and, using a fork or potato masher, allow it to cook while you mash the beef to keep it from clumping together until slightly browned.
5. Add the tomato paste, coconut aminos or soy sauce, and 1 cup of water. Let the mixture simmer for 15 minutes over medium heat.
6. Turn off the heat and, if necessary, add more salt and spices to taste.
7. Serve with a squeeze of lemon over the cooked macaroni.

Easy Lamb Meatballs

MAKES 4 SERVINGS

Calories: 260
Protein: 23 grams
Carbohydrates: 2 grams
Fat: 17 grams

These tender and flavorful lamb meatballs are packed with protein and healthy fats, making them a satisfying and nutritious meal option. With just a handful of ingredients and minimal prep time, you can create a delicious dish that's perfect for a quick weeknight dinner.

Ingredients

1 pound ground lamb
2 tablespoons plain Greek yogurt or dairy-free yogurt
2 garlic cloves, minced
1 teaspoon sea salt
1/2 teaspoon pepper
1 teaspoon onion powder
1 teaspoon ground cumin
1 teaspoon ground cinnamon
1/2 cup chopped curly parsley, plus more for serving
2 tablespoons extra-virgin olive oil
1 lemon, sliced, for serving

Instructions

1. Place a rack in the middle of the oven. Preheat the oven to 375°F.
2. In a large bowl, mix the lamb, yogurt, garlic, salt, pepper, onion powder, cumin, cinnamon, parsley, and olive oil together.
3. Using a 1 1/2-tablespoon cookie scoop, scoop out even portions of the mixture onto a plate.
4. With wet hands, shape each portion into a round meatball and set on a baking sheet. Bake for 15 to 18 minutes, until slightly brown.
5. Serve with fresh lemon slices and additional parsley.

Coconut Butter Salmon with Roasted Vegetables

MAKES 4 SERVINGS

Calories: 450
Protein: 40 grams
Carbohydrates: 25 grams
Fat: 20 grams

Not only is this recipe quick and easy to make, it's packed with protein and healthy fats and is a great way to get your daily dose of vegetables.

Ingredients

1 tablespoon extra-virgin olive oil

1 teaspoon salt

½ teaspoon pepper

¼ teaspoon fresh lemon juice

1 pound salmon fillet, skin on

1 tablespoon coconut butter

1 head of broccoli, cut into florets

2 carrots, peeled and sliced

1 zucchini, sliced

Instructions

1. Preheat the oven to 400°F. Line a baking sheet with parchment paper.
2. In a small bowl, combine the olive oil, salt, pepper, and lemon juice.
3. Rub the mixture all over the salmon fillet and place it on the baking sheet. Crumble the coconut butter evenly over the salmon and arrange the broccoli, carrots, and zucchini around it.
4. Bake for 20 to 25 minutes, or until the salmon is cooked through and the vegetables are tender.
5. Serve immediately.

Gluten-Free Chicken Stir-Fry

MAKES 2 SERVINGS

Calories: 400
Protein: 30 grams
Carbohydrates: 40 grams
Fat: 15 grams

This recipe is a great way to get your daily dose of vegetables, and it's also a good source of protein.

Ingredients

1 tablespoon extra-virgin olive oil

Salt

1 pound boneless, skinless chicken breasts, cut into bite-sized pieces

1 onion, chopped

2 carrots, peeled and sliced

1 head of broccoli, cut into florets

1 teaspoon minced ginger

2 garlic cloves, minced

1/4 cup coconut aminos

1/4 cup chicken broth

Instructions

1. In a large skillet or wok, heat the olive oil over medium heat.
2. Lightly salt the chicken pieces and add them to the skillet. Cook the chicken, stirring occasionally, until browned on all sides.
3. Add the garlic, onions, carrots, broccoli, and ginger, and cook until the vegetables are tender-crisp.
4. In a small bowl, whisk together coconut aminos, chicken broth, and 1 tablespoon of water. Add the mixture to the skillet and cook until thickened.
5. Serve immediately over rice.

One-Pot Arroz con Pollo (Chicken and Rice)

MAKES 1 SERVING

Calories: 490
Protein: 25 grams
Carbohydrates: 70 grams
Fat: 12 grams

An easy one-pot arroz con pollo (chicken and rice) dish cooked with flavorful spices, onions, and peppers. This dish is ideal for batch cooking and great as leftovers if you wanted to make enough to last a few days.

Ingredients

4 garlic cloves, minced
1/2 teaspoon paprika
1/2 teaspoon ground coriander
1/4 teaspoon dried oregano
1/4 teaspoon ground cumin
1/4 teaspoon sea salt, plus more to taste
6 ounces boneless, skinless chicken thighs, diced
1 tablespoon extra-virgin olive oil
1 sweet onion, chopped
1 green bell pepper, chopped
3/4 cup rice or quinoa
Broth (how much depends on the amount of water whichever grain you choose requires to cook)
2 tomatoes, chopped
Black pepper to taste
2 tablespoons chopped fresh cilantro, for serving
1 lime, sliced, for serving

Instructions

1. In a medium bowl, combine the garlic, paprika, coriander, oregano, cumin, and salt. Remove half of the spice mixture and set aside.
2. Add the chicken pieces to the first bowl of spices and toss to coat.
3. In a large skillet, heat the olive oil over medium heat. Add the onions and bell peppers and cook until lightly browned.
4. Add the rice or quinoa and the reserved spices and stir to combine for about 30 seconds. Add the broth and tomatoes, mixing it up really well.
5. Bring it all to a boil. Add the chicken and reduce the heat to low. Cover and simmer for about 15 minutes, or until the rice or quinoa is tender.
6. Remove from the heat and let rest for 10 minutes.
7. Before serving, season with salt and pepper and garnish with the fresh cilantro and lime.

Chocolate-Beet Smoothie

MAKES 1 SERVING

Calories: 300
Protein: 15 grams
Carbohydrates: 40 grams
Fat: 15 grams

This smoothie is a great pre-workout choice because it provides a balance of fat, protein, and carbs. The beets and cacao powder also add a few health benefits, including improved blood flow and increased endurance.

Ingredients

1 cup chopped frozen bananas

1/4 cup diced cooked beets

1 tablespoon cacao powder

1 tablespoon chia seeds

1 date, seeded

1/2 cup unsweetened almond milk

1 scoop chocolate protein powder (optional)

1 shot espresso (optional, for extra energy)

Instructions

Combine all the ingredients in a blender and blend until smooth.

POST-WORKOUT SMOOTHIE

Strawberry-Cherry Recovery Smoothie

MAKES 1 SERVING

Calories: 300
Protein: 20 grams
Carbohydrates: 40 grams
Fat: 10 grams

Cherries have many antioxidant and anti-inflammatory polyphenol compounds that accelerate strength recovery after exercise. The protein powder in this smoothie helps to build and repair muscle tissue, while the carbohydrates restore energy to the body.

Ingredients

1 cup frozen strawberries

1 cup frozen dark cherries

1/2 cup unsweetened almond milk

1 scoop vanilla protein powder

1 tablespoon ground flaxseeds

1 teaspoon chia seeds

1/2 teaspoon ground cinnamon

Ice, to taste

Instructions

Combine all the ingredients in a blender and blend until smooth.

Cherry Chocolate-Chip Walnut Granola Bars

MAKES 6 OR 7 BARS

Calories: 210
Protein: 3 grams
Carbohydrates: 31 grams
Fat: 9 grams

Know exactly what's in your pre-workout granola bar with this recipe using whole ingredients.

Ingredients

1¼ cups gluten-free rolled oats

⅔ cup walnuts

½ cup dried cranberries, chopped

½ cup raw sunflower seeds

¼ cup Enjoy Life semi-sweet chocolate chips

½ teaspoon sea salt

½ teaspoon ground cinnamon

2 tablespoons almond butter

½ cup dried dates, pitted and soaked in warm water

Instructions

1. In a food processor, pulse the oats, walnuts, cranberries, sunflower seeds, chocolate chips, sea salt, and cinnamon until combined and broken up into smaller pieces.
2. Add almond butter and dates. Pulse until the mixture forms a paste and starts to stick to itself, likely forming a ball.
3. On parchment paper, spread out the ball and cut it evenly to form 6 or 7 bars.
4. Chill to firm up and store the bars in the fridge.

Grain-Free Blueberry Muffins

MAKES 12 MUFFINS

(TAKE THESE UP A NOTCH WITH EXTRA PROTEIN BY ADDING ONE SCOOP OF YOUR FAVORITE COLLAGEN POWDER.)

Calories: 190
Protein: 4 grams
Carbohydrates: 25 grams
Fat: 5 grams

Ingredients

3 cups Bob's Red Mill paleo baking flour

1 tablespoon ground cinnamon

1 teaspoon baking soda

1/2 teaspoon salt

4 scoops protein powder of choice

3 eggs

3/4 cup melted coconut oil

1/2 cup honey

3/4 cup fresh blueberries

Lemon zest, for garnish

Instructions

1. Preheat the oven to 350°F. Line a 12-cup muffin tin with paper liners.
2. In a medium bowl, combine the paleo baking flour, cinnamon, baking soda, salt, protein powder, and any upgrades you would like to add; set aside.
3. In a large bowl, whisk together the eggs, coconut oil, honey, and 1/3 cup water.
4. Add the flour mixture to the eggs and mix thoroughly. Stir in the blueberries.
5. Spoon the batter into the prepared muffin tin. Bake for 20 to 25 minutes. Use a toothpick test: Stick a toothpick into the muffin and pull it out. If it comes out clean, they're done.
6. Remove the muffins from the oven and add lemon zest over the tops.
7. Let the muffins cool in the tin before you enjoy.

Garbanzo and Cashew Hummus Dip

MAKES 1 SERVING (2 TABLESPOONS)

Calories: 80–100
Protein: 2 grams
Carbohydrates: 3 grams
Fat: 5 grams

A twist on a classic favorite dip! Adding cashews gives your hummus an elevated creamy texture you are sure to love. Use the spice recommendations here as a starting point, but have fun by playing with the measurements to find your winning combination.

Ingredients

- 1 cup cooked chickpeas, drained and rinsed
- 1/2 cup cashews, soaked for 10 minutes and drained
- 1/3 cup smooth tahini
- 2 tablespoons extra-virgin olive oil
- 2 tablespoons fresh lemon juice, plus more to taste
- 1 garlic clove
- 1/2 teaspoon salt, plus more to taste
- 1/4 teaspoon cumin, plus more to taste

Instructions

Blend all the ingredients together with 5 tablespoons water, adding up to 5 more tablespoons of water until the dip is silky smooth. Taste the dip and, if necessary, add additional lemon juice, salt, and cumin to taste.

Serving suggestions: Eat with fresh veggies and a protein on low-performance days and with extra carbs, such as crackers or pita bread, on high-performance days.

Simply Stuffed Dates

MAKES 1 STUFFED DATE

Calories: 112
Protein: 3 grams
Carbohydrates: 12 grams
Fat: 10 grams

Don't overthink it.

Ingredients

1 date, split open and pit removed

½ tablespoon almond butter

1 almond

Instructions

Stuff the date with the almond butter and top with the almond for a bit of crunch.

PART II

MOVE

CHAPTER 7

Think It Forward

Does age play a role in holding back your body? To a certain extent, sure. But no matter what you think or what you've been told, it's not inevitable that as time passes we all sort of just fall apart. If we become weaker, less mobile, and more injury prone with age, it isn't just Father Time's fault.

It's ours.

As we age, most of us become less active and neglect to do preventative maintenance—and yet we expect our body to perform just as it did decades ago. We quite literally *will* ourselves to feel, move, and act older than we really are because of three major mistakes:

1. We write ourselves an IOU. For one, the older we get, the more responsibilities we take on, and that performance slide most people see in their thirties and forties tends to happen because some of the time we would typically put into ourselves gets channeled into other important pursuits. The thirties and forties are our prime earning years, so we feel pressure to take professional advantage of that block of time, take more risks, burn the midnight oil. If you're a parent, the time you have for yourself gets divided even further, juggling parental duties among everything else.

How do we cope with all these extra duties? We make a deal with ourselves, sacrificing our health *now* and promising we'll get back our old self *later*.

I'm not saying any of those priorities are wrong. Having a great relationship with your spouse and kids and knowing you can retire comfortably are admirable goals. But in order to truly enjoy the *later*, you still have to invest in the *now*, especially when it comes to mobility.

2. We focus on the wrong M. When you were in your twenties and thirties, did you even give a second thought to longevity? Did you do any extra exercises with an eye toward injury prevention?

Of course not. Most of us, when we're young, take our bodies and what they're capable of doing for granted. You probably warmed up your body or stretched only if it was cold that day or when told to by a coach, because for the most part, you could always rely on it to perform at a moment's notice. Sure, the chances of pulling a muscle or hurting yourself were always there, but not bothering with preventing that from happening was always worth the risk.

When working out, most people focus on their *muscles*, but their first priority should be on their *mobility*. Simply put, they pay attention to the wrong M. Spend too much time and effort on only trying to forge stronger, leaner muscles and you risk creating muscular imbalances that increase your chance of injury and curtail your full range of motion.

However, when you concentrate on improving your mobility by incorporating certain key stretches and exercises, you can roll back the clock to those days when you felt invincible. This regimen will keep your joints, ligaments, and secondary supportive muscles more pliable and resilient, preventing injury, and will also allow them to contribute to other exercises. It will get all of your muscles working as they were intended to—in synchronicity with one another—making you not only more flexible, but also stronger and faster.

3. We never evolve our exercise. I often see people stick with (or return to) workout routines from when they were younger. They reminisce about what they used to be able to do and assume that whatever worked years ago will give them that same level of functional fitness. But the thing is, our bodies change, and every few years, we must change the way we do things. If you're not twenty-one anymore, then you need to stop exercising exactly like you did when you were twenty-one—only then do you have a shot at feeling twenty-one again.

LeBron doesn't train the same way he did when he was twenty-five years old. Sure, there are certain strength-training exercises we've always used to improve different aspects of his game, certain drills that maintain his strength and stamina to help him continue to be an all-around player. But to keep him on the court—to keep his career going for as long as possible—we've had to evolve his routine to match his body. Now it's more about fluidity and resilience. That's where my mobility method comes in.

What to Think Through . . .

Before Starting This Program

What Are You Bringing to the Table?

What I mean is, how active are you—really? What is your daily routine and how long have you been doing it? And has that daily routine been in place for the last week? The last month? The last year?

Clients come to me at different stages, from beginner to advanced, from sports professionals looking for an athletic edge to others of average health just looking to finally have a body that feels and functions better.

No matter what sport or activity you're already involved in, or how you typically choose to exercise, or, heck, whether or not you're even active at all, this program will take you to a higher place than you are right now—because it prepares your body—*any* body—to perform and live up to its maximum potential.

If you're an athlete or exercise regularly. You and I both know that you're the type of individual that already takes ownership in their body, so know this: My routine isn't meant to replace whatever you're doing right now—it's designed to complement it. I'm solidifying the foundation of the house you've already built so that nothing knocks you down.

If you're worried that incorporating my routine will lead to overtraining, then put your fears to rest. The entire program utilizes low-risk movement exercises that can be dialed back if needed, but the sum effect should be the opposite of overtraining. Instead, you'll notice improvements in your activity of choice in both your productivity and energy level.

If you're presently inactive. Even if you've never stepped foot into a gym or played a sport in your life, you will become a more biomechanically efficient human being. Within just a few sessions, you will feel and move better than ever before as you gain mobility, become stronger, and develop more stamina in the portions of your body that matter most, including your spine, lower back, core, and other key muscles, joints, and ligaments. Each day, you're going to get more from every movement you make from sun up to sundown.

That said, doing *only* my program—even if it makes a huge impact on your life—isn't the life you deserve. That's why in the next chapter, I'm going to suggest a few ways you can find moments throughout the day to move more.

Are You *Truly* Ready for This?

If this is your first time attempting my functional program, then know there's a mindset that needs to be in place.

1. Be prepared to stay awhile. Some of these moves may be familiar to you, but I know that others won't be. It won't take too long to familiarize yourself with each move and seamlessly flow from one to the next, but it's not going to happen overnight. So be patient, trust the process, and know that you'll become faster with practice.

2. Get ready to feel sore. Even though many of the moves I'm encouraging you to do daily are stretches, there are just as many movements that are strength and/or endurance-building exercises—and you'll feel them the next day. And the day after that. But that's a good thing! What you're experiencing is known as "delayed onset muscle soreness" (DOMS), inflammation triggered by the tiny, microscopic tears in your muscles that occur as you exercise, as well as a buildup of excess lactic acid, the waste product left behind in your muscles after they break down sugar (glucose) to generate adenosine triphosphate (ATP) for energy.

You will likely feel the sorest in your abdominals (the abs) and your posterior chain muscles (the muscles on the backside of your body, particularly your calves, hamstrings, glutes, erector spinae muscles, and upper/lower back). Because most people focus on their "mirror muscles" (those they can see in the mirror), the posterior chain muscles don't typically see the same volume of effort as they deserve.

The good news is, DOMS is only temporary. And because some of the movements are stretches, you may not feel as sore from the buildup of lactic acid as you might expect. You see, whenever you stretch a muscle, your body responds by increasing the flow of blood to that area. With that blood comes additional oxygen, which helps remove excess lactic acid, lessening the chances you'll be sore the next day.

3. It's about inches–not miles. Having just a little more mobility will make a huge difference in your daily performance—but don't expect to see huge visual differences. Being able to reach just another few centimeters farther in a particular stretch or having the endurance to hold a certain posture for a few more seconds more can and will make a significant improvement in how well your body functions all day long—even if that progression seems slight to you at first.

What Time *Really* Works for You?

Ideally, I want you to do my mobility regimen first thing in the morning because I believe your day should always start with project number one—and that's you.

When you start the day by investing in yourself, you'll immediately begin to see dividends. If that makes you feel selfish, it's important to remind yourself how taking care of yourself first actually helps everyone around you because you'll be more able physically to take care of them as well. You'll be more energetic and flexible throughout the day, in addition to having your core left in a more engaged posture. It leaves your body primed and ready for anything.

On top of the physical benefits, you'll also be starting the day with the mindset of knowing that you've already accomplished one of the most important tasks you can do for your body. Once this is off your plate before your day even really begins, it psychologically prepares you by reminding you what you're capable of. It instantly becomes an example you can reflect on throughout your day during moments when you might think you don't have the ability to put enough time or energy into your job, your family, others around you, or yourself.

However, you need to be enthusiastic when you put in the effort. If that's not possible because you're just not a morning person, don't try to force a square peg into a round hole. I mean that sincerely. I would rather you do this routine when it's convenient for you *if*—and only if—that's what it takes to keep you 100 percent invested. If it's only possible for you to do it right after lunch, once the kids go to bed, or random times each day because you're never sure when you'll have a moment to yourself, so long as you're giving me—so long as you're giving yourself—all your energy and focus, then go ahead.

Another reason I don't have a problem with you squeezing in the program whenever is best for your schedule is this: Once you begin to feel its effects, as you begin to notice how much better your body feels afterward, you may find yourself waking up a few minutes early to do it in the morning because you want to experience that feeling all day long.

What's the Worst Day This Week?

I usually meet with LeBron first thing in the morning because he's a morning person and he brings the energy every single time. But during our years together, there have been a handful of times when he won't say a word—and I can tell something is bothering him. My main concern those days is getting him to a better place. What I've found works is not, as you might think, pulling back the volume of work to make things easier—but, rather, pushing him to make things as hard as possible. Because afterward, every single time, he feels so much better and realizes that he has more energy—energy to take on whatever was on his mind before we began.

So many people are prepared to do what it takes physically, but few are prepared to do what it takes mentally. Could that be you? One quick way to find out is to inconvenience yourself early into starting my program to see how you handle adversity when it comes to exercise. I'm not asking you to do anything extreme here, but what I'm encouraging you to try—if you're serious about doing this program long-term—is to look ahead at your week, pick the busiest day, and then make sure that on *that* day, you make the time to do this routine. I'm talking whichever day you're expecting to have to juggle a million things—and make a commitment to start the day with this program, no excuses.

I want you to do this for several reasons: First, because it proves to yourself that it **is** possible to carve out enough minutes for yourself and this program, despite the demands of that day. It puts the hardest day of the week in your rearview mirror, which makes it impossible to blow off doing the routine on days that are less stressful. But most important, it's a reminder of what you're capable of, so if something comes out of left field—if suddenly a day that was supposed to be smooth sailing becomes chaotic and you don't think you can manage squeezing in this program—you'll know that you can, because you have a history of doing it.

Another reason I want you to do this is because it will help you tackle that stressful day with more energy. And, if there is something pressing on your mind or bothering you on that day, don't be surprised if you'll feel that the problem is less of a big deal, or perhaps you'll walk away with a breakthrough epiphany, saying to yourself, "Man, I'll fix it that way! I get it now!"

These are big promises, I know. I can preach the routine's benefits all day long, but until you experience it for yourself, you'll never be absolutely sure that it does work. But when you intentionally commit yourself to do the program on your worst possible day—I'm not saying every week, but every once in a while—it reinforces the fact that doing it every day will put you in a better place, no matter how tired or stressed you may be. So that way, the next time you find yourself debating whether to do the plan when things get busy, you'll be less likely to skip the session because you'll remember how much better you'll feel and think afterward.

Does Your Attire Inspire?

This is a program designed to enhance mobility. I also want you to really dial into how your body is feeling throughout each movement, which can sometimes be hard to do if what you're wearing is so constrictive that it distracts you. For that reason, your clothing must allow you to bend, twist, or stretch comfortably.

As for footwear, the very first movement requires your shoes to be off to stretch your plantar fascia (the band of tissue that runs from your heels to your toes). After that, your first instincts might be to throw on a pair of cross-trainers or some other footwear for stability—but, if possible, don't.

Ideally, if you can kick your shoes off and keep them off (and you're not breaking any rules by doing so), I prefer you stay barefoot—otherwise you'll lose a portion of the proprioceptive benefit of the workout. Going shoeless also improves the communication between what's above you and below you, since your feet relay information to your brain regarding how stable you are, how much force is being placed through each leg into the ground, and other vital details of body awareness.

What to Think Through . . .

Before Every Mobility Session

How Do You Feel in *This* Moment?

You'll never know how far you've gone unless you know where you've been, right? That's why before you even attempt not just this routine but any physical activity, it's important to take an honest inventory of yourself. You need to preassess how you feel right before you jump into the routine and give yourself a quick head-to-toe, inside and out—what I call a "body baseline."

Don't worry, this won't hurt. All I want you to do is answer five questions about yourself, the same five questions I'd be asking you if I was about to put you through the paces in person. Why do you need to do this?

- You'll be less likely to injure yourself because you'll be listening to your body *before* it embarks on whatever you're about to ask of it.
- You'll also make a stronger connection with the program because when you answer these same questions afterward, when it's time to "break down" the program, you will not only see and feel how your body is moving more efficiently, but also notice how the answers change in a positive way. The more often you recognize the program's effectiveness, the more likely you are to stick with it and see lifelong results.

This self-diagnosis need not be perfect. If you're not quite sure if something feels sore or can't decide whether your energy is at a five or a seven, don't overthink it. Just be honest. That means no hiding behind your pride.

The more genuine you are answering these questions, the more you're going to grow from this program. That goes for every time in this book that I ask you for an honest assessment. Now, let's get started:

Copy this page for convenience (in fact, make a few because you'll need them), then circle/write your answers prior to and every time you perform my mobility program.

1. **Do you feel sore in any of these areas (circle all that apply)?**
   Feet. Ankles. Calves/Achilles. Hamstrings. Quadriceps. Hips. Midsection. Lower Back. Upper Back. Shoulders. Arms. Neck.
2. **Do you feel tight/stiff in any of these areas (circle all that apply)?**
   Feet. Ankles. Calves/Achilles. Hamstrings. Quadriceps. Hips. Midsection. Lower Back. Upper Back. Shoulders. Arms. Neck.
3. **Do you feel weak in any of these areas (circle all that apply)?**
   Feet. Ankles. Calves/Achilles. Hamstrings. Quadriceps. Hips. Midsection. Lower Back. Upper Back. Shoulders. Arms. Neck.
4. **Where would you rank your energy level?**
   (1 being the least alert; 10 being the most alert):
   1 2 3 4 5 6 7 8 9 10
5. **Where would you rank your motivation?**
   (1 being "just phoning it in"; 10 being "ready to crush this"):
   1 2 3 4 5 6 7 8 9 10

Are You Feeling Unsure This Is All Worth It?

Each time you complete my program, you will feel a difference that will carry out through your day and improve all aspects of your life. But if you're looking for a more obvious example that illustrates its effectiveness—or ever feel any lingering doubts—I want you to do what I call the **Four Before**.

Prior to doing my mobility program, try performing each of the following four movements just a handful of times. Pay attention to your balance and coordination as you do each of them—in fact, record yourself with your phone if you want so that you have something to look back on.

Then, after completing the entire mobility program, run through each of these movements once more. The difference between the "before" and "after" might seem slight, but how more fluidly and efficiently you move should be easily detectable.

1. **Single-leg stork stance:** Bend your right leg and bring your right knee up in front of you so that your right thigh is parallel to the floor and you're balancing on your left leg. (Your hands can remain on your hips.) Hold for as long as possible, then switch positions so that you're balancing on your right leg for as long as possible.
2. **Heel raise:** Stand up straight with your feet together and arms down at your sides. Raise your heels up as high as you can and balance on your toes for as long as possible.
3. **Single-leg reach and grab:** Imagine you're a golfer about to take your ball out of the hole. Balance on one leg and reach down to touch the ground, letting the opposite leg extend behind you. Switch positions to work the other leg.
4. **Bodyweight squat and hold:** Stand straight with your feet hip-width apart and your arms extended straight above your head (upper arms in line with your ears). Squat down until your thighs are almost parallel to the floor and hold for as long as possible.

Okay, enough talking about moving—let's get moving!

CHAPTER 8

Follow It Through

Let's rip the Band-Aid off right now.

There is no one-size-fits-all program that answers the needs of everybody—or should I say every *body*. Not everything that works perfectly for one of my clients will work perfectly for you, and that's normal.

Let me put it another way: Even world-class athletes on the same team don't typically train the exact same way. Instead, they often train in a specific way to improve a set of skills or certain muscle groups that may need more work, or to rehab other areas that require a little extra downtime. When I meet with a client, I look at what they need to get from their body at that specific moment, and then I tailor my plan to those demands.

But underneath every program I put together is a foundation of functional strength and flexibility movements. This set of exercises and stretches works like a launchpad, helping them soar farther and faster, no matter which direction they're heading.

I'm about to share with you that foundation—the principal movements that not only LeBron does, but all my clients who share the same all-encompassing goal of moving forward as far as possible for as long as possible. It's a program designed to help your body function at a much higher level than it is presently by combining the smartest forms of movement. This series of stretches and exercises will prepare your body to perform at its highest possible level while simultaneously minimizing your risk of injury.

Why This Plan?

Your body is a machine, specifically designed to move in a precise way. When allowed to operate as intended, your body is capable of far greater things than you could ever imagine. But when it's kept from doing its job—when we don't repeatedly remind our body how it was meant to move—it learns a series of bad habits that can negatively impact every single movement you make.

Right now, your body spends most of its time supporting itself in positions it was never meant to be placed, such as sitting down hunched over a computer or phone. The more off-center your spine is due to poor posture, the more difficult it is for you to function at your best.

Whenever I see a golfer up at the crack of dawn at the first tee, I laugh. You'll see them stretching to limber themselves up at 6:30 Saturday morning because their tee time is at seven. But then Monday comes, and that same golfer just rolls out of bed, has a cup of coffee, and goes straight to work instead of activating their body before attacking the day.

Shouldn't you care as much about your life as you do your handicap? Isn't how you move throughout the day, no matter how ordinary you may think those movements are for the next sixteen or so hours, worth preparing for? We'll take the time to do certain functional movements to improve our game, our score, our reps and sets, our performance, but we won't take the time to do certain functional movements to improve our day in general. In other words, we will take the time to prepare our bodies for an event or a sport, but we don't do it for daily life. The problem with that mentality is that longevity isn't just about being a more agile athlete in the moment—it's about being a more agile individual all day long. That's where my twenty-seven-move mobility and core stabilization program takes over—let's call it my "mobility regimen" for short.

My mobility regimen is a simple, uniquely balanced head-to-toe program that works your body both from an athletic-training standpoint and a physical-therapy perspective. This program doesn't just increase your mobility and strengthen your core—it reminds your body of its own mechanics.

The more you practice it, the more you'll not only be engaging and stretching the muscles most people ignore or never consider (such as the plantar fascia, calves, toes, and hip flexors), but you'll be reteaching your body how it should be positioned during specific movements. Your body will quickly begin to automatically stabilize itself more effectively and eliminate unnecessary steps as you move, allowing you to perform any task—whether in the weight room, in sports, or in everyday life—with the least amount of effort and fatigue. In addition:

- This routine uses certain functional moves that teach your upper and lower body to better utilize your core muscles, which equates to more speed, power, and balance when moving in any direction.
- It creates a stronger core that helps your body divide stress evenly, making it more effective at absorbing shock.
- It keeps your joints, ligaments, and secondary supportive muscles strong and healthy, allowing them to contribute more to every move so you can lift more weight with less risk of injury.
- It keeps your spine in line by preventing tight lower back muscles or a weak core from pulling it out of its natural alignment—a mechanical imbalance that can create neck and back problems and cause your muscles to fatigue faster.
- It recruits your proprioceptive muscles, a series of neurological stabilizers that make slight tweaks to your posture all day long to keep your body in alignment.
- Finally, it keeps the muscles you see in the mirror from sidelining you. Most people typically have stronger anterior muscles (the muscles in front of you) than posterior muscles (the muscles behind you), a battle of wills that can make you more susceptible to impingement problems, tendonitis, and other movement-related injuries down the road. This routine helps prevent any muscular imbalances caused from overdeveloped muscles pulling against weaker ones from impacting your performance or getting you hurt.

The Rules of the Regimen

The twenty-seven movements I want you to do fall into three categories:

- **The Six-Pack of Stretches**—The first six movements are all stretches that you will do from a seated or standing position.
- **The Core On-the-Floor Fourteen**—For the next fourteen movements, I'm bringing you down to the ground. You'll be lying down, kneeling, or in a position closer to the floor for all fourteen.
- **The Stand-to-Command Finale**—For these last seven strength-building movements, you'll be returning to a standing position before I see you off for the day.

(By the way, just because I've divided the routine up into three specific sections, that doesn't mean you should pause between each one.)

Some of these movements might be familiar, while others will likely be foreign to you. But collectively, they create a complete head-to-toe package specifically aimed at maximizing your overall performance. They help you forge a more functional body that will lengthen your longevity and make you less prone to injury, but only if you do them as instructed.

Where to Do It

Even though many of my clients have access to state-of-the-art equipment, due to their travel schedules they often find themselves in situations in which access isn't always possible, making it harder to stay consistent. That's why I build regimens with accountability in mind using minimal equipment, so it's easy to stay the course no matter where you find yourself.

This program requires no equipment whatsoever. You can do it at home, in a hotel room when traveling, even in your office if you have some free time between meetings. But find a place where you feel comfortable. If comfortable for you is in front of your TV watching the morning news, or in a room far away from family, with candles lit and soft music playing, then so be it—so long as you're able to listen to your body, be aware of every movement, and connect with how each one is making your body feel and react.

But seriously, a place with minimal distractions is best because this is *your* time, and these movements are an investment in yourself. If you try to do them on a morning conference call or any situation where you can't focus on them, you'll only be cheating yourself.

How Often

Unlike many programs that might expect you to work out five days in a row (with weekends off) or have some other sort of rigid structure that might not sync up with your life, my routine doesn't take that sort of cookie-cutter approach.

If someone comes to me and says that they already work out five days a week, I might tell them to do my routine three times a week (Monday, Wednesday, and Friday), or each day they exercise (five days total), or if they're active and their schedule can handle it, I might even encourage them to do an abbreviated version of my routine Saturday or Sunday morning on top of those five days. It really depends on the individual. But here are some broad-stroke recommendations:

For the inactive: If you're new to exercise or currently sedentary, I want you to start with **two days on/one day off**. That means perform the regimen two days in a row, then take the third day off. (For example, if you're starting at the beginning of the week, do it Monday and Tuesday, then take Wednesday off.)

After that, see how you feel. When I work with folks that aren't used to pushing themselves mentally and physically, two days in a row is a big win, and then they often need one day off to rest (and celebrate their accomplishment) before getting at it again.

Another variation you can try is **three days on/two days off**. Again, for example, if you start at the beginning of the week, you will go Monday through Wednesday, then take Thursday and Friday off (starting the next three-day cycle on Saturday).

For the active: If you currently exercise (or work a physically demanding job) at least three days a week, you have options as well. You could:

- Try a **three days on/one day off** schedule, performing my regimen whenever you wish (on days you're active or inactive).
- You could **do the routine only on days that you're active**, so long as you're active at least five days a week. If you're active less often than that, then you might end up doing the regimen less each week than I'm asking of beginners.

No matter what your present activity level, at some point, you're going to know when you can step it up and try a schedule of:

- **Four days on/one day off**
- **Five days on/one day off**
- **Six days on/one day off**

For my overachievers: If you're inclined to do the program seven days a week, then you're in rarefied air—because I don't even ask my high-performance clients to do that. Seriously, I want to be out of your head for at least a day every week because I never want you thinking, "Oh, man, I have to do Mike's program today."

It's not just that I don't want you to hate me. It's that you won't progress that much further by doing that extra day. Instead, allowing yourself one day of rest from the program each week will keep you from mentally burning out, which ultimately will lead to you sticking with the program for life.

With Every Exercise and Stretch

Go in order. You'll start with Movement #1, then perform all twenty-seven movements in the *exact order* shown—one after the other with no rest in between (minus the time it takes you to get yourself into each new position).

However, when I say no rest, I don't mean rush yourself through the workout. Once you finish a movement, move on to the next at a normal pace.

Breathe with purpose. That means inhaling through your nose and exhaling through your mouth. Holding your breath—or breathing erratically—during certain strength-training movements will only deprive your muscles of oxygen, as well as potentially elevate your blood pressure.

Don't worry about the numbers. You're going to notice that I'm not requiring you to do that many repetitions of each movement. That's for several reasons: One, because you're addressing your entire body with a variety of multi-angle movements, there's no reason to go overboard with repetitions. And two, more repetitions just makes most people feel they need to get it over with—they just want to check off the box that says "done" at any cost—and that can lead to rushing through the regimen. Each of these twenty-seven moves is about quality, not quantity. You'll get more bang for your buck doing fewer repetitions with better form than more repetitions done hastily and sloppily.

Know that a little bit still counts. If you're not able to move as freely as you'd like with certain movements, do what you can and do not get discouraged. You might not have the range or flexibility right now, but it will come soon enough.

In the meantime, whenever you find you can't move as freely as you'd like, or stretch as far or as deep as you think you should, or lack the strength or endurance for any movement—get excited! Because whenever I see that lack of ability in a client, I also feel excited. I know then that that person has been living with a deficit for who knows how long—possibly their entire life up until that moment—which means they're about to realize their untapped potential.

What if a particular movement feels either too easy or too difficult? All twenty-seven movements can be modified to either be more manageable or elevate their intensity. If you run into any issues as you experience the regimen for the first time—or later as your body begins to adapt to it—just turn to Chapter 10 to learn how to adjust each one to your current fitness level.

Finally, it's twenty-seven movements—and no fewer. What's imperative is that you do each and every one of these movements for the allotted time—no exceptions or substitutions. There is a reason behind all these movements and how long (and often) you should be doing them.

Look, I know it might seem like a lot of steps, but many of these movements seamlessly flow into one another, which minimizes setup time in between. It's also a reminder of how you should be approaching your entire day, not shying away from demanding situations just because you struggle with them. With life—as with this routine—you must take the good with the bad, and try to engage with the difficult bits if you want to grow.

Common Questions My Clients Ask

Am I going to need a lot of equipment? Nope. All of the exercises within the regimen are bodyweight movements, so for now, there's no weights or strength-training equipment required. All you'll need to get started is yourself, a chair (or a place to sit), a wall you can lean against (for a few select movements), and a tennis ball (for the first exercise). However, one thing I do recommend investing in is an exercise or yoga mat. Certain stretches and exercises will have you positioned on the floor, so having a softer but supportive surface will make these movements more comfortable.

How long will the regimen take? I find that most clients finish the entire regimen around the twenty-minute mark. That may sound like a lot to some people, and if that's you, remind yourself that within that window, you are literally preparing your body performance-wise for the entire day. If twenty minutes seems like a lot of effort to reap all the benefits that LeBron and my other clients have experienced over the years, stop asking, "Why does it have to take so long?" and instead ask yourself, "Isn't living my best life—being able to move and function at the highest level possible—worth spending a few minutes on myself?"

Should I warm up my body beforehand? That's entirely up to you. The routine itself is going to warm up your muscles (which is why I just mentioned how it could be used as a warm-up prior to exercise or activity). But if you want to wake up your muscles before you use them, feel free to lightly jog in place for three to five minutes.

Could I do this twice a day? If you have the time to do so, absolutely. You could do it in the morning and either repeat it after work, in the evening when you're relaxing, or right before bed. In my opinion, if you're considering twice a day—and it's possible for you to do so—I would do that second session after lunch, right at that spot in the midafternoon when most of us hit a lull, because if your mind is in that state, your body isn't far behind.

Could I use the mobility regimen as a warm-up/cool-down? Yes. Just as the full routine prepares you for the entire day, it's possible to use a shortened version of my program as a warm-up/cool-down prior to or immediately after a workout, game, or anything physical. In fact, LeBron does an abbreviated version as a range of motion warm-up before performing certain strength-, speed-, and muscle-building routines he also does to improve his game. I don't have to worry about his form or technique performing any exercise because doing that shorter version of my routine primes and preps his body, especially his core, for activity.

So how would you go about shortening this? The easiest way is to run through all twenty-seven movements in the exact order given but do each exercise/stretch for one-third to half the time (or repetitions) suggested. For example, if I told you to do a move for six to eight repetitions, do it only three to four times. If I suggested holding a pose for twenty seconds, hold it for ten instead.

What I don't want you to do is eliminate any movements, cherry-pick your favorites, or just stop halfway through to shorten things up. All twenty-seven movements prepare your body from the ground up, and they all work together to improve performance. If you ever think of taking that route instead of what I've recommended, please remind yourself of the reason you're using a shortened routine in the first place: You're attempting to warm up your body to lessen your risk of injury and perform at your best. Every movement you choose to skip leaves certain muscles tighter and less activated. Why would you put your body in that compromised position?

Now, could you also use the entire program as prescribed as a warm-up without shortening it? For example, if you typically run at noon and wanted to use my routine to warm yourself up prior to lacing up your shoes and hitting the street? Or, if you only have time to exercise in the evening, or if after work is when you get together with your team and play? The answer is yes, but it really depends on how much time you have and what your body is capable of. So long as you never feel as if you're pushing your body too hard to the point where you feel your performance is negatively impacted, feel free to go for it.

Wait—Didn't I Just Do This Move?

Throughout this routine, you're going to see what looks to be slight variations of certain exercises or stretches that you literally just did seconds before. That's by design, because with certain movements, it's important to bring your body up to speed before you expect big things from it.

Think about it this way: If you were going to bench-press your max, would you start by lifting as much weight as possible—or would you build up to it by using less weight and then adding plates? If you were going to sprint as fast as humanly possible, would you simply step onto the track right out of the locker room and take off—or would you warm up your muscles first?

Some of the movements within this routine require more coordination, stability, flexibility, and strength than others. More important, they require a stronger mind-body connection. That's why you'll notice that certain stretches or exercises build off one another. In many cases, whatever movement you just did prepared you for the movement you're about to do. And the movement you're about to do is, well, preparing you for the movement you'll be doing directly after that.

Pain—Temporary or Troublesome?

Having you assess your pain level might sound like a big ask—I mean, you're not a doctor, right? Well, neither am I, but you don't have to be one to pinpoint warning signs that you should heed.

Experiencing some muscle soreness during or following my program is perfectly normal, but if you notice any pain that's either sharp or burns, stop the routine immediately and have yourself seen by a doctor to be safe. This goes double if that pain is focused on a bone or joint.

For the record, none of my twenty-seven movements should be the cause of the pain, but even the safest of movements can sometimes reveal underlying issues that need to be addressed.

The Six-Pack of Stretches

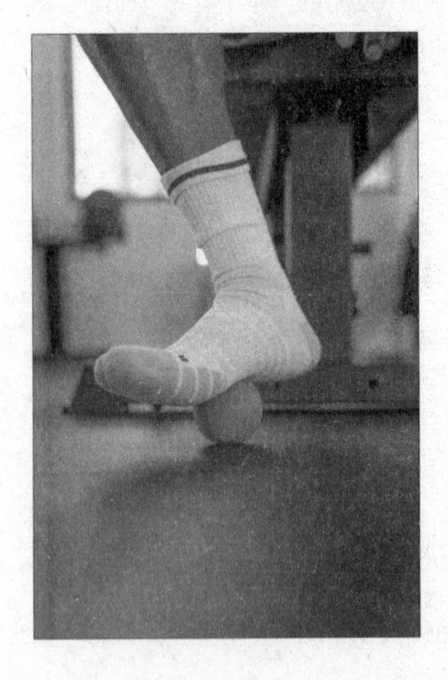

1. Plantar Fascia Stretch

What it's working [Loosens and activates your plantar fascia—the connective tissue on each foot between your toes and heel]

Ready? Sit on a chair—or the edge of your bed—and place a tennis ball on the floor by your feet. Step on top of the ball with one foot.

Set . . . Gently press down so there's a slight amount of pressure from the ball pushing up into your foot.

Go! Slowly roll the ball back and forth from your heel to your toes. (If you're not currently experiencing any issues with your feet, go 30 seconds. But if you are presently experiencing plantar fasciitis, stick with rolling the ball for 60 seconds.) Once finished, switch the ball to your opposite foot and repeat.

The Difference Maker

- Don't just roll the ball backward and forward along the same path. Try to shift the ball to the left and right to work the entire bottom of your foot.

Why it's essential: I start this program—and every program—by waking up the feet. They may seem inconsequential, but they're the two major players responsible not only for supporting your weight but deciding how effectively you stand, walk, jump, and run.

Stability starts with your feet and how well they respond to the ground. If your feet aren't in tune with the rest of your body, then you're automatically a little bit off center and imbalanced. That's why you need to stretch out the muscles and wake up the neural sensors within them.

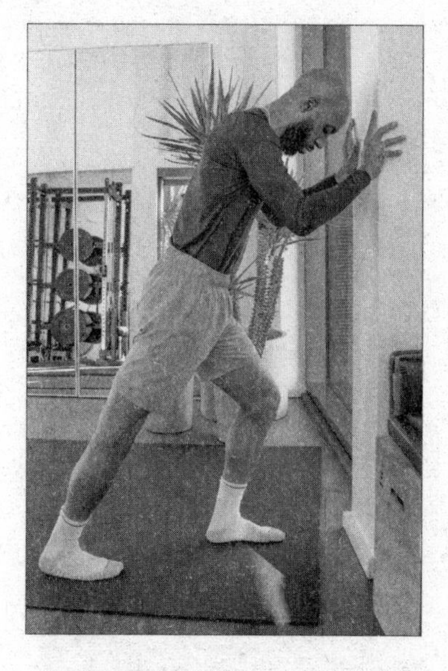

2. Standing Wall Stretch

What it's working [Loosens the calf muscles and the Achilles tendon]

Ready? Stand facing a sturdy wall and place your hands flat against it. Position your legs in a split stance, left foot several feet in front of your right foot, toes facing forward.

Set... Make sure your feet are flat on the floor from heel to toe.

Go! Bend your left knee until you feel the stretch within the lower leg muscles of your right leg, then return to the Set position. Do the move for 10 to 12 repetitions, then switch positions—placing your right foot several feet in front of your left foot—and repeat the stretch with your left leg.

The Difference Makers

- Don't just keep your back heel flat during this stretch, but actively try to press it into the floor.
- Resist the urge to arch your back. Keep it as straight as possible.

Why it's essential: Calf-muscle strains are one of the most common injuries athletes (from amateur to elite) suffer from, which is why showing your lower legs a little love with this stretch is so important. But another reason is that it also limbers up the Achilles tendon in each leg, the strongest tendon in your body, which connects your heel bone to your calf muscle and comes into play every time you rise on your toes. By regularly keeping this tendon more pliable, you can help prevent it from becoming inflamed, which can lead to Achilles tendonitis, the root cause of most ankle and foot pain.

3. Standing Hamstring and Nerve Floss Stretch

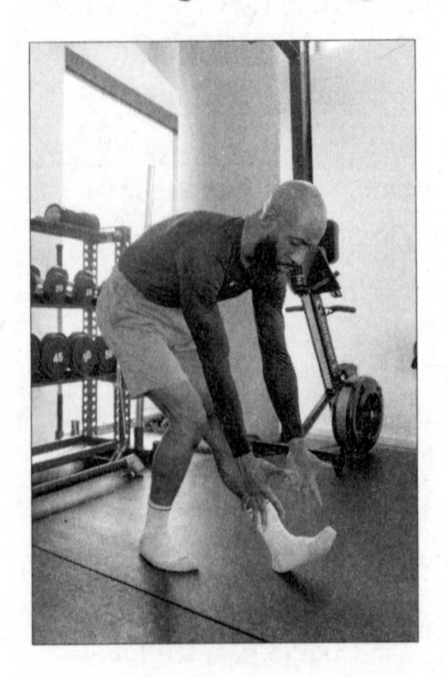

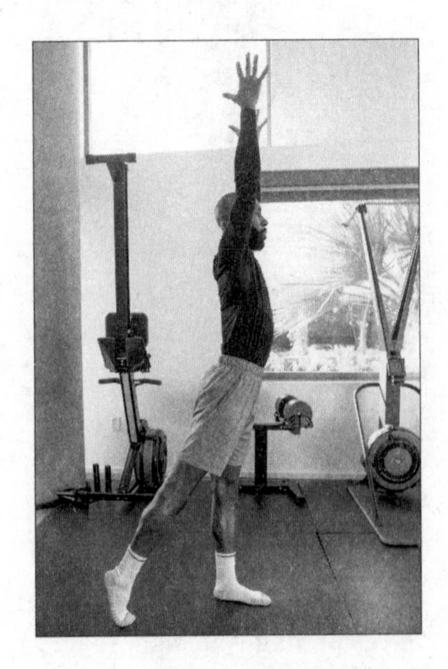

What it's working [Loosens the hamstrings—the upper leg muscles located in the back of your thighs—and flosses your sciatic nerve]

Ready? Stand in a split stance—legs straight, left foot several feet in front of your right foot, toes facing forward.

Set... Raise your arms up over your head, palms facing each other.

Go! Once you have your balance, slowly bend forward from the hips—not your back—as you simultaneously sweep your arms downward and lift the toes of your left foot up off the ground. Raise yourself back up into the Set position and do 6 to 8 repetitions. Switch positions—this time placing your right foot several feet in front of your left foot—and repeat.

The Difference Makers

- Try not to round your back—it should stay as flat as possible the entire time. The movement isn't about how far down you can go but feeling the stretch within your hamstrings.
- Engage your core by contracting your abdominals. This trick also makes it more difficult to round your back.

Why it's essential: Most people are walking around with tight hamstrings, which makes this stretch a mainstay in my book. However, a lot of people are also walking around with asymptomatic herniated discs. (I'm not kidding when I say that could be you right now—it's that common.) That's why it's so important to stretch the nerve that literally controls pain, discomfort, and numbness in the lower back and the legs.

Even if your back feels fine now, you still might have underlying nerve issues that can flare up at any time. Worse still, you never know what kind of position you're going to be in when it does flare up. Will it happen when you're lifting something heavy? Could it occur at a moment that might put you at a greater risk of injuring other parts of your body at the same time? By adding this simple stretch, you'll not only keep your hamstrings nice and loose, but you'll minimize your chances of experiencing any sciatic nerve issues over time.

4. Alternating Quad Stretch

What it's working [Loosens the quadriceps, the upper leg muscles located in the front of your thighs. It also teaches you how to engage your core to maintain balance]

Ready? Stand straight with your arms down by your sides.

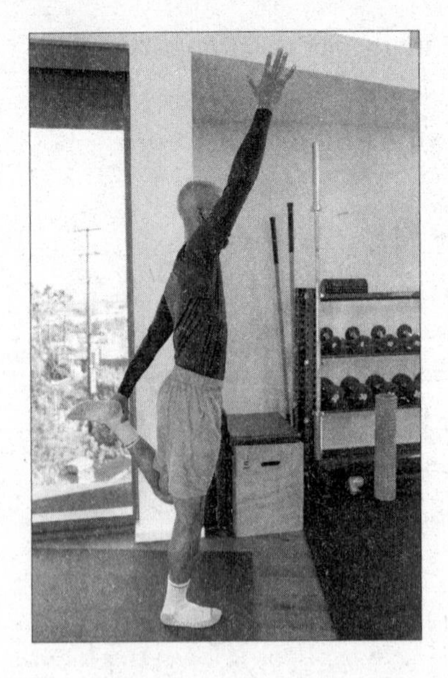

Set . . . Bend your left knee and raise your left foot up behind you toward your butt. Reach back with your left hand and grab it. Finally, extend your right arm upward.

Go! Gently pull your left heel toward your butt, hold for 2 seconds, then let go and let your left foot return to the floor. Next, repeat the move by bending your right knee and raising your right foot up. Catch it with your right hand, extend your left arm upward, pull your right heel toward your butt, hold for 2 seconds, then release it. Continue to alternate from left to right for a total of 10 repetitions (5 for each leg).

The Difference Makers

- Try not to hold on to anything. This stretch challenges your proprioceptive muscles and improves your balance, but only if you avoid grabbing something for support.
- Take your shoes off if possible. By performing this exercise barefoot, you also work all the tiny intrinsic muscles within your feet that supportive shoes typically shut down.

Why it's essential: A pair of tight quadriceps creates muscular imbalances that can make you more susceptible to knee and lower back pain, as well as injury elsewhere. That's why keeping them as loose as possible is so critical for performance.

The reason I prefer this more active way of stretching your quadriceps is that you're always moving instead of just standing there, which simultaneously improves your reflexes when you're unstable. You're also indirectly strengthening your quadriceps and glute muscles of whichever leg you're balancing on to support your weight.

The good news is, even if you lose your balance and need to catch yourself occasionally, you're still not failing. What you're indirectly doing is training your reflexes by teaching your body to react as quickly as possible when unstable, a reaction that transfers over into real life and can help minimize the odds of injuring yourself in sports, at work, at home, etc. (So don't kick yourself for losing your balance trying to "kick yourself"!)

5. Single-Arm Pectoral Stretch

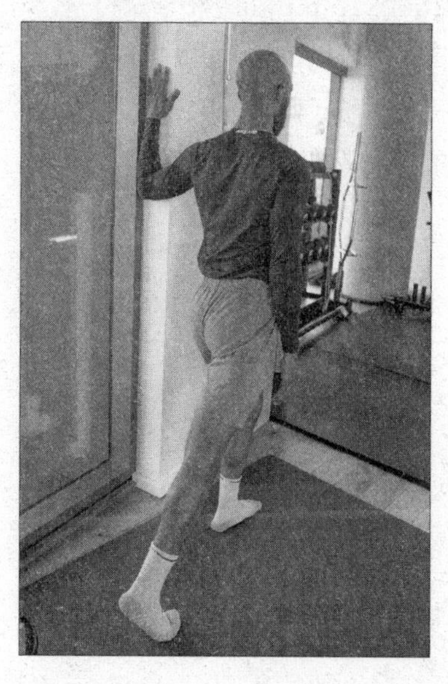

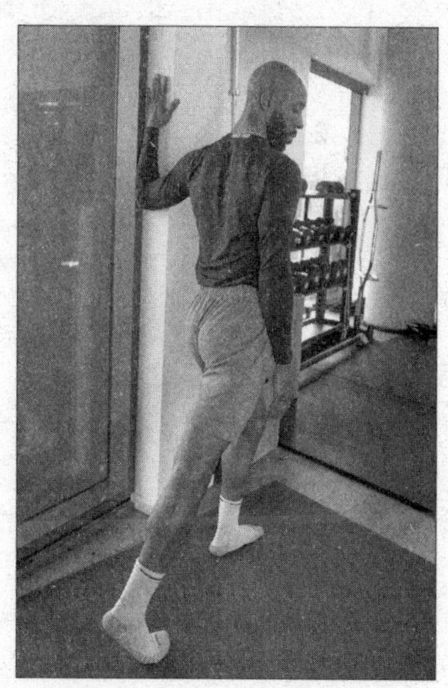

What it's working [Loosens the muscles of the chest (both pectoralis minor and major), shoulders (primarily the anterior deltoid), and neck]

Ready? Stand in front of an open doorway as if you're about to enter it. Get into a split stance (left foot forward, right foot back) and position yourself so that your shoulders are in line with the doorway.

Set... Bend your left arm at about a 90-degree angle, raise it out to your side (fingers pointing up and your upper arm parallel to the floor), and place your left hand flat along the left side of the doorway. Your lower arm from your fingers down to your elbow should rest along the doorway.

Go! Keeping your left arm on the wall, step forward as far as you comfortably can until you feel a slight stretch along the outside of your chest. As you go, turn your head to the right until you feel a stretch and look down.

Hold for 3 to 5 seconds, then change positions to perform the stretch with your right arm. (This time, place your right foot forward, left foot back, and turn your head to the left before looking down.) Alternate from left to right 8 times (4 repetitions per arm).

The Difference Maker

- Breathe as deeply as you can as you hold the stretch to really open up your pectoral muscles.

Why it's essential: Very rarely do you find someone with great posture and an open chest, particularly because most of us suffer from postural issues caused by excessive technology use. We spend a disproportionate amount of time bowed-over looking down at our phones or computers, leading to poor posturing that negatively affects the muscles within the chest. That's why everyone can benefit from this slightly modified version of a classic chest stretch.

Constant technology also takes its toll on your neck. When your head is positioned down, your trapezius—the long, triangle-shaped muscle that attaches at the base of your skull and connects to the back of your collarbone and shoulder blades—is kept tight instead of remaining supple and loose. Also, very few people perform a lot of rotational stretching movements (looking side to side) into their day, so this stretch helps to relax your neck and trapezius muscles to increase your range of motion and minimize pain.

6. Angel Stretch

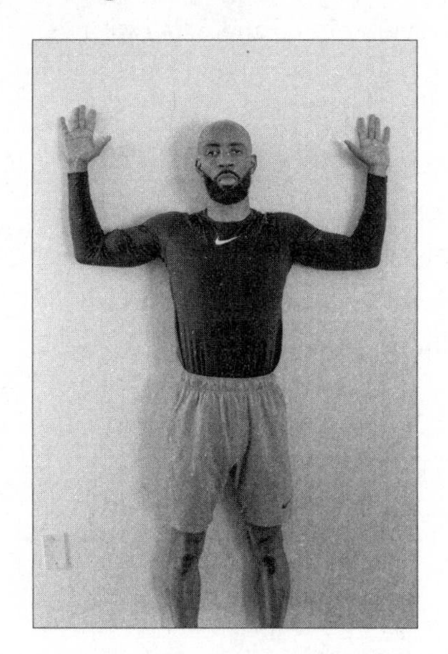

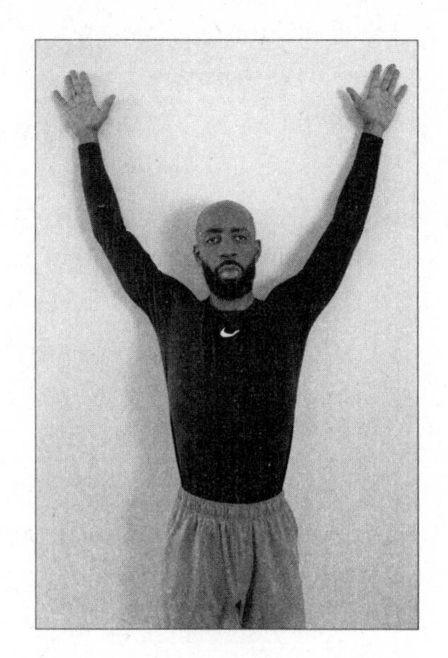

What it's working [Loosens up the latissimus dorsi, pectorals, shoulders, and postural muscles]

Ready? Stand with your back facing a wall, feet hip-width apart. Raise your arms up as if someone just said, "Stick 'em up!" Your arms should be bent at the elbow with your hands roughly in line with your head, palms facing forward.

Set . . . Flatten yourself up against the wall so that your head, upper back, elbows, the backs of your hands, butt, and heels are all touching the wall. None of them should lift off the wall throughout the entire exercise.

Go! Slowly slide your arms up and out until your arms are straight and at 45-degree angles to your body—if you've done it right, you'll look like the letter Y. Slide your arms back into the starting position and do 8 repetitions.

The Difference Makers

- Ideally, take 3 to 5 seconds to raise your arms up and 3 to 5 seconds to lower them down.
- As you go, engage your upper-back muscles by squeezing (contracting) them.
- If you ever feel your body not touching the wall in the places I've mentioned, that means your posture isn't as straight as it should be, so immediately fix it. When you have better posture, all those body parts stay in contact with the wall with less effort and require less concentration.

Why it's essential: This exercise not only opens up the rib cage and expands your lungs, but it simultaneously works to strengthen and straighten your postural muscles.

The Core On-the-Floor Fourteen

Time to bring things to the floor, so grab your exercise/yoga mat and drop down for these next few movements.

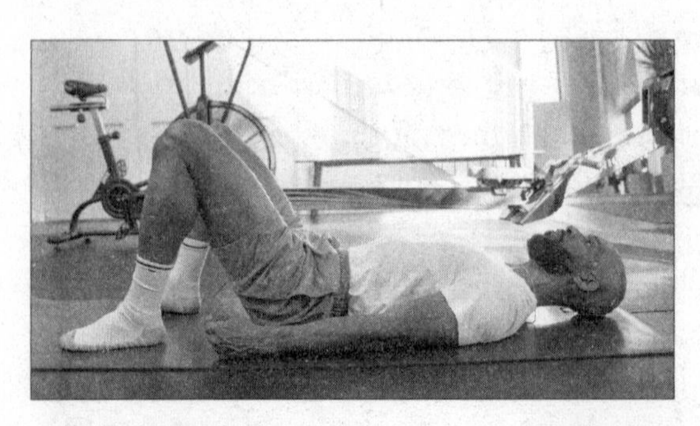

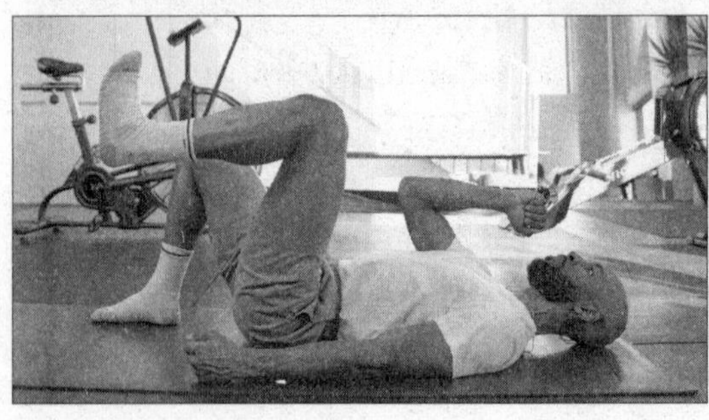

7. On-the-Floor Marching

What it's working [Strengthens your core muscles and hip flexors]

Ready? Lie flat on your back with your arms positioned straight along your sides. Bend your knees so that your legs are bent at a 90-degree angle.

Set . . . Make a pair of fists and turn your palms in toward you. Tighten your core muscles and prepare yourself to keep them engaged throughout the entire movement.

Go! Keeping your head flat on the floor, slowly bend your left leg and raise your left knee up as you simultaneously bend your right arm and swing it up. At the top of the movement, your leg should be bent at about a 90-degree angle (with your thigh perpendicular to the floor).

Return to the Set position and repeat the movement, this time slowly bending your right leg and raising your right knee up as you simultaneously bend your left arm and swing it up. Shoot for 20 repetitions total (10 for each side).

The Difference Makers

- Don't be tricked by the word *march* into doing this one quickly. Going too fast only creates momentum that can shift you out of proper alignment and rob you of the movement's benefits. I want you moving at a very slow and controlled pace that keeps you in touch with your breathing.
- Think of a moderate drum rhythm in your head—then follow that beat. A good pace to try: Before you do the move, count Mississippis and tap your hand on your leg as you say each number (ONE Mississippi, TWO Mississippi, THREE Mississippi, etc.). The beat that you're tapping is a perfect place to start, rhythm-wise.
- Avoid watching your knees work. Being curious about what's going on down there only compromises your breathing. Instead, I want your chin up so that you're staring directly at the ceiling.

Why it's essential: Having a strong core, good posture, and proper spinal alignment is central to everything. This simple exercise effectively works on all three, which is why I like to call it "the queen bee of the hive."

With it, you're not just strengthening specific postural muscles. It also turns your midsection into a tighter cylinder that makes other movements—whether in sports or daily activity—much more efficient and less prone to injury. It literally teaches your core how to stabilize itself during motion so that later in the day, whether you're lifting weights or just picking up your kids, your spine is always protected.

8. On-the-Floor Pilates 100

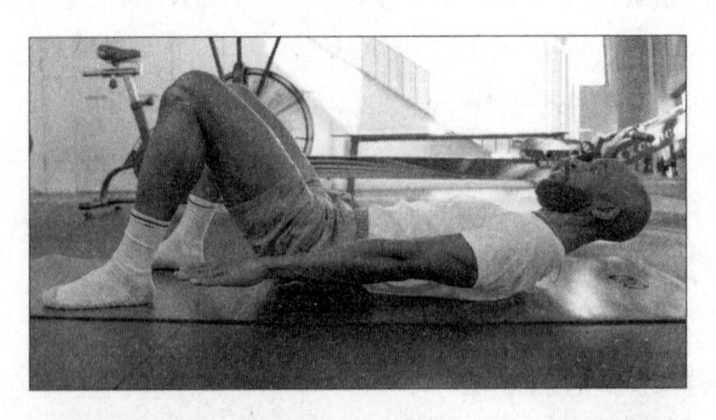

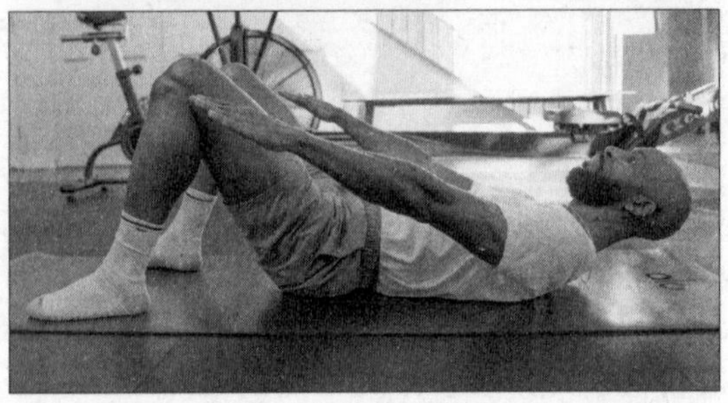

What it's working [Strengthens your lower core muscles, shoulders, hip flexors, and latissimus dorsi]

Ready? Lie flat on your back with your arms straight down at your sides, palms facing down. Bend your knees so that your legs are bent at a 90-degree angle.

Set... Next, raise your head and neck up off the floor. Raise your arms up so that your hands are about 6 inches from the floor.

Go! Keeping your head and legs up and off the floor, begin pulsing your arms up and down for 50 repetitions. Rest for 30 seconds, then perform another set of 50 repetitions.

The Difference Makers

- Focus on not moving anything except for your arms.
- Try not to touch the ground with your hands but get as close as possible.
- Don't hold your breath as you go. Inhale through your nose for a count of 3 to 4 seconds, then exhale with your lips pursed (as if you're blowing out a candle) for 3 to 4 seconds.

Why it's essential: What I love about this move is that it never puts anything at risk. A lot of abdominal exercises require you to flex at the spine, which, if not done exactly right, can stress your lower back. This is a very functional core movement that engages the entire body without putting your spine in a compromising position.

9. Glute Bridge

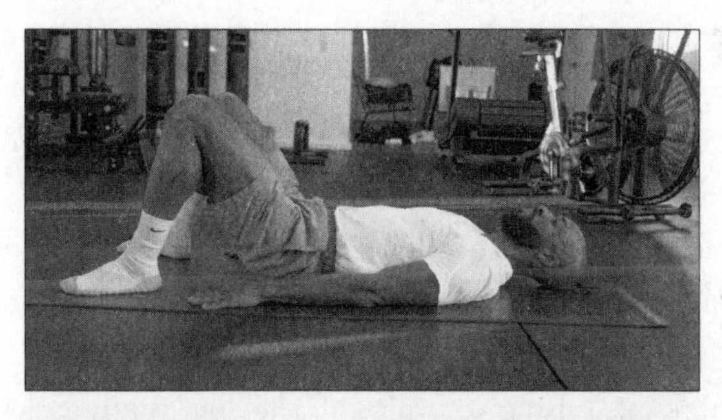

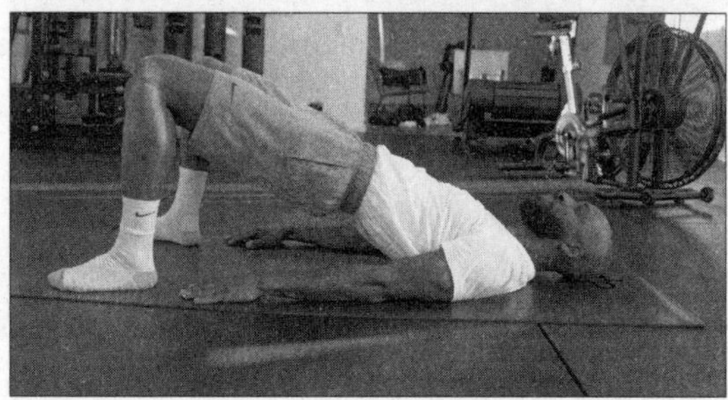

What it's working [Strengthens the gluteus muscles—primarily the gluteus maximus—as well as the hamstrings (the muscles in the back of your thighs) and the transverse abdominis, a thin sheet of abdominal muscle essential for stabilizing the core and spine]

Ready? Lie on the floor face up with your knees bent and your feet flat on the floor, hip-width apart. Your arms should be down at your sides, palms facing down.
Set... Pull your stomach in, gently contract your core muscles, and hold this posture throughout the entire movement.
Go! Contract your gluteal muscles and raise your hips upward until your body forms a straight line from your knees down to your shoulders. Pause for 3 seconds, then lower yourself back down into the Set position. Repeat the move for 10 to 12 repetitions.

The Difference Makers

- Concentrate on driving your heels into the floor before and as you rise.
- Resist the urge to curl your neck up to watch your body lift up. Instead, keep your head flat on the ground at all times.
- Don't let your butt just drop back down to the floor. Stay in control by resisting gravity on the way down.
- Don't dismiss the "contract your glutes" portion of the exercise and think just raising your hips off the floor is just as good. By doing so, you'll maximize glute activation while simultaneously minimizing your risk of discomfort in your lower back and/or hamstrings from cramping.

Why it's essential: The glute bridge isn't just a fantastic, no-equipment-needed way to strengthen your glutes, but it's easily one of the most vital movements often overlooked in most strength and body maintenance programs. It not only promotes better posture and balance, decreases back pain, and improves core strength, but it also elevates your athletic performance by helping to stabilize your posterior chain, allowing you to tap into more leg strength and stability, as well as overall power when making explosive movements.

Back to your butt for a second. This move is the first of other movements within my routine that target your gluteus maximus (one of the strongest and biggest muscles in your body), gluteus medius, and gluteus minimus—the three muscle groups that make up your glutes. Whenever you walk, run, squat, bend, lunge, or twist, your glutes come into play, which is why they ultimately decide how far you can improve your posture, balance, and overall strength during any activity. Considered one of the most important muscle groups for total athleticism, they serve many roles when it comes to movement, from producing and reducing force from your hips, stabilizing your body as you change direction (especially during side-to-side motions), and generating rotational power whenever you swing or throw—just to name a few.

10. Push-Up

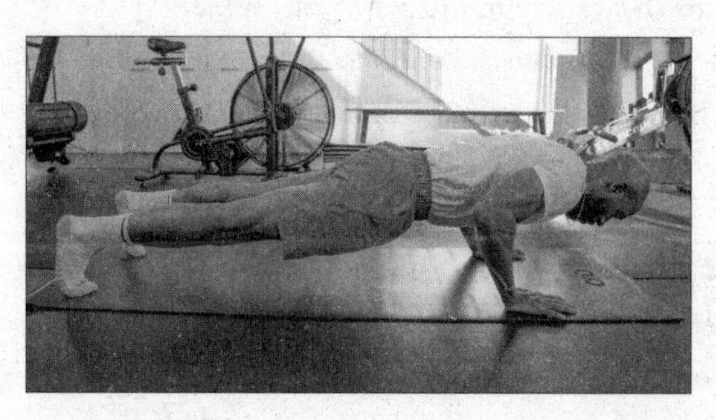

What it's working [Strengthens your chest, shoulders, and triceps, as well as your core muscles]

Ready? From a kneeling position, place your hands flat on the floor (shoulder-width apart), keeping your arms straight, elbows locked. Extend your legs straight behind you with your weight on your toes (or the tops of the balls of your feet).

Set... Align yourself so that your hands are directly below your shoulders—your arms should be perpendicular to the floor. Finally, pull in your stomach and contract your core muscles.

Go! Slowly bend your elbows and lower yourself down until your upper arms are parallel to the floor. Push yourself back up until your arms are straight, elbows unlocked. Perform 8 to 15 repetitions.

The Difference Makers

- Tuck your upper arms (and elbows) as close to your sides as possible—if they flare out, you're placing unnecessary stress on your elbows.
- Don't rush the movement. Take 2 seconds to lower yourself down and 2 seconds to push yourself back up.
- Look straight down at the floor and resist the urge to turn your head to the side or tuck it to see your feet. Your head and neck need to always stay in line with your spine.
- Keep your core muscles contracted the entire time. This prevents your hips from dropping and helps position your body in a straight line from your head down to your heels.

Why it's essential: The push-up, of course, is a classic. This multi-muscle movement is incredible at triggering the natural release of HGH (human growth hormone) and is primarily known as a complete upper-body exercise, which it is. But it's also an incredible tool for teaching your core how to work with the muscles above it.

You see, it takes proper core initiation to get yourself up off the ground during a push-up. That's because a strong core helps keep your body in alignment, allowing your chest, shoulders, and triceps to work more efficiently together to push you up and lower you down. But when your core isn't strong enough to maintain your posture, your chest muscles must step in and help. The problem is, they're designed to push (not stabilize your center), so they end up wasting energy they could be using to help push you up and away from the ground. By mixing this classic move in with other core exercises—instead of just doing it during a regular workout—it reminds your muscles how they're designed to work together to get the job done.

11. Bent-Knee Side Plank

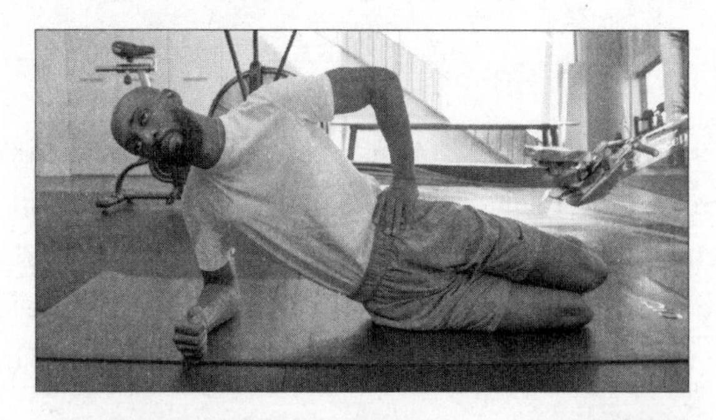

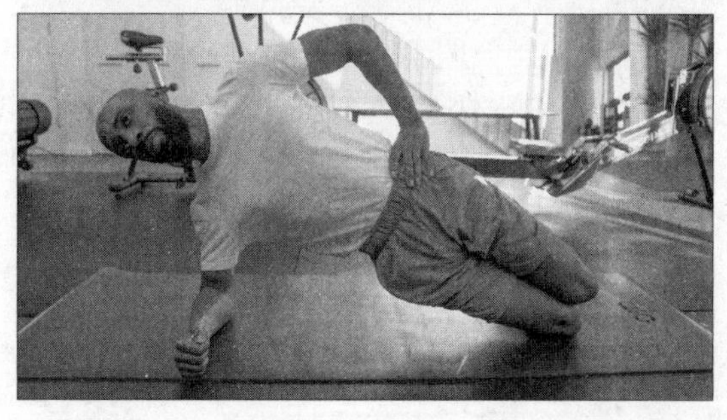

What it's working [Strengthens your glutes, hips, and core muscles]

Ready? Lie down on your right side with your legs straight and prop yourself up on your right elbow—your right arm should be bent at 90 degrees with your fist pointing directly in front of you. Your left hand can rest on your left hip. Finally, keeping your knees stacked on top of each other, bend your legs 90 degrees so that your feet are behind you.

Set . . . To prevent any extra compression in your shoulder, make sure your right elbow is always directly underneath your right shoulder. Avoid looking down at your knees and instead look straight ahead.

Go! Slowly push down through your elbow and raise your hips up until your body forms a straight line from your head to your knees. Pause for 5 seconds, lower your hips back down, and repeat 5 times. Afterward, switch positions by lying on your left side and repeat the exercise.

The Difference Makers

- Tighten your core muscles and keep them contracted throughout the entire movement.
- Contract your glutes and keep them contracted throughout the entire movement. This will automatically keep your pelvis pushed forward, which prevents your hips from flexing as you raise up.

Why it's essential: When you do it right, you're strengthening your glutes (for superior leg power) and it's conditioning your obliques (love handles) and core muscles. Collectively, all these muscles work together to protect your lower back from injury.

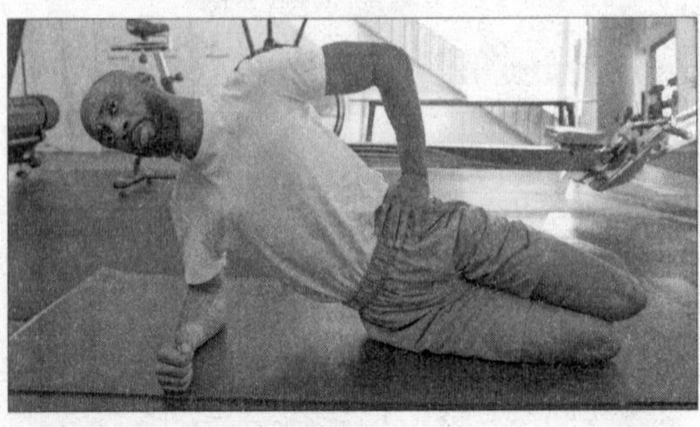

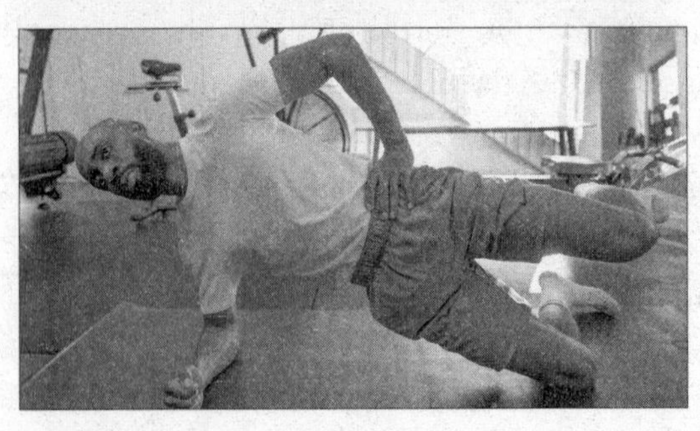

12. Side Plank with Leg Raise

What it's working [Strengthens your glutes, hips, and core muscles, as well as your adductors]

Ready? For this variation, you'll get into the same position as the Bent-Knee Side Plank. Lie down on your right side with your legs straight and prop yourself up on your right elbow—your right arm should be bent at 90 degrees with your fist pointing directly in front of you. Your left hand can rest on your left hip. Finally, keeping your knees stacked on top of each other, bend your legs 90 degrees so that your feet are behind you.

Set... Slowly push down through your elbow and raise your hips up until your body forms a straight line from your head to your knees.

Go! Holding this position, raise your left leg up as high as you comfortably can, then lower it back down (but don't let your knees touch, if possible). Do 8 to 12 repetitions, then switch legs for an additional 8 to 12 repetitions.

The Difference Makers

- Move at a comfortable pace, but not so fast that you lose your balance. You want to stay in control of the exercise the entire time. Ideally, shoot for 3 seconds up and 3 seconds down if possible.
- Don't let gravity do the work for you. Stay in control of your top leg as you lower it.
- Because you're moving your top leg, it's easy to forget that what's equally important is keeping your body in a straight line, so don't let your hip drop.

Why it's essential: When you do a traditional side plank, the glute on the bottom is the one primarily doing most of the work keeping you supported. But adding a leg raise forces both sides to activate at the same time in addition to your adductors (a series of muscles within your inner thigh that brings your legs together). These small but highly important muscles are often hard to train but are crucial for maximum hip mobility and strength.

13. Side Plank March

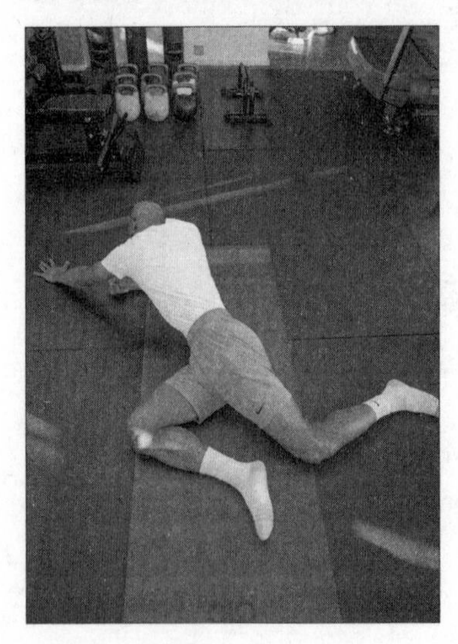

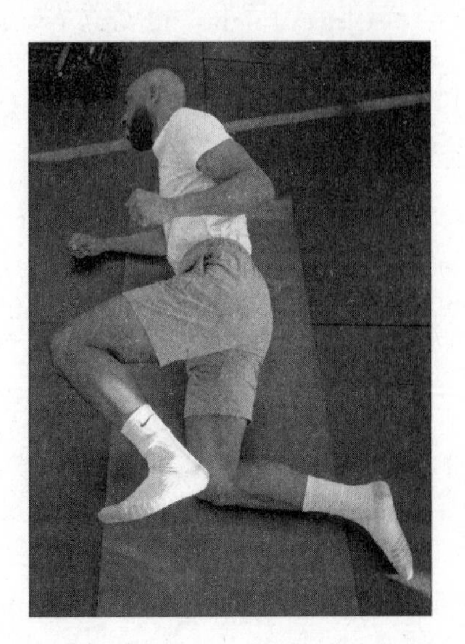

What it's working [Strengthens your glutes, hips, obliques, and core muscles]

Ready? Lie down on your right side with your legs straight and prop yourself up on your right elbow—your right arm should be bent at 90 degrees with your fist pointing directly in front of you. Bend your right leg 90 degrees so that your right foot is slightly behind you, right knee slightly forward.

Set . . . Place your left leg (knee bent) behind you and bring your left arm in front of you. From a bird's-eye perspective, you should look like you're almost in a running position.

Go! Slowly push down through your elbow and raise your hips up until your body forms a straight line from your head to your knees. As you come off the floor, simultaneously swing your left leg in front of you (keeping your knee bent) while swinging your left arm back behind you. Reverse the motion by lowering your hips back down to the floor as you simultaneously swing your left leg back behind you and your left arm in front of you.

Repeat 8 to 10 times, then switch positions to work your right leg for an additional 8 to 10 repetitions.

The Difference Maker

- Again, move at a comfortable pace that doesn't cause you to lose your balance. But for this one, you can move at a slightly faster pace than the Side Plank with Leg Raises, so think 2 seconds up and 2 seconds down.

Why it's essential: This is the finisher that puts the last two side plank versions together, working your upper body, lower body, and core in unison. It will also improve your overall shoulder stabilization because you'll be pivoting off your shoulder and bottom knee. This movement is more dynamic than the Side Plank with Leg Raises, so while it's working the same muscles, it will feel just a little bit harder.

14. Traditional Plank

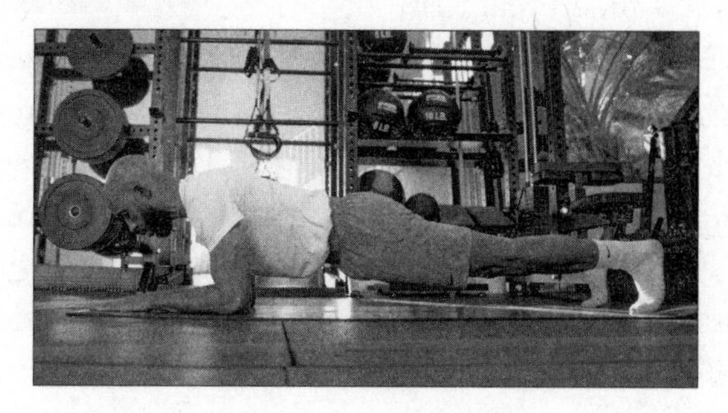

What it's working [Strengthens your core muscles, particularly the rectus abdominis (the six-pack muscles) and transverse abdominis, as well as—to a certain degree—your lower back, trapezius, rhomboids, chest, quadriceps, glutes, and calves]

Ready? Get down on the floor into a push-up position, placing your hands about hip-width apart and your legs extended straight behind you, feet together. Next, bend your arms and rest on your forearms with your palms flat on the floor. (Your elbows should be directly below your shoulders.) Finally, position your neck in line with your spine—your eyes should be facing straight down at the floor instead of looking forward or to the side.

Set... Pull in your stomach, then contract your core muscles—and keep them like that the entire time. Imagine having to tighten up your stomach as if someone was going to punch you in the gut. Your body should form a straight line from your heels up to your head.

Go! Hold this position for 15 to 20 seconds.

The Difference Makers

- To help keep your torso even straighter, lock your shoulder blades by gently pressing your elbows down into the floor as you simultaneously push your upper back upward and shift your shoulders toward your feet.
- To keep your hips from dropping, contract your glutes.
- Watch your base. Placing your forearms or feet wider than hip-width apart will only make it easier to balance and rob you of results.

Why it's essential: Placing this universal movement at the midpoint of the routine sort of resets the table. It's a wake-up call to your core to stay tight so that it's primed and ready to stabilize you for the movements that are about to come.

15. Superman

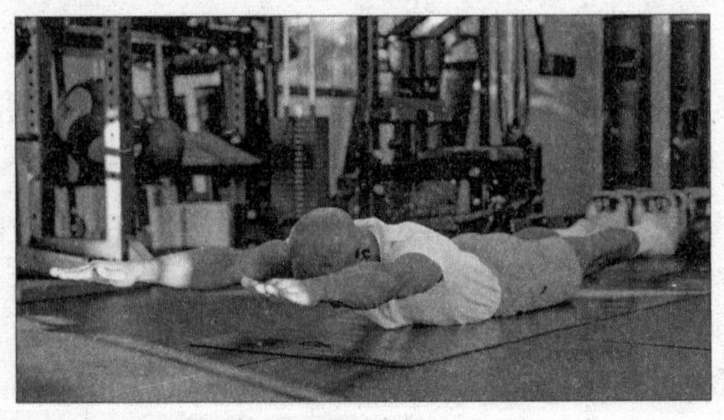

What it's working [Strengthens your lower back, hamstrings, glutes, upper back, shoulders, and abdominals]

Ready? Lie face down on a mat (or any surface soft enough to cushion your pelvis) and extend your arms and legs. Your body should form a straight line from your fingertips to your feet.

Set... Turn your hands so that your palms are facing the floor, then pull your toes inward toward your knees so that you're resting on your toes (not the tops of your feet). Finally, position your head and neck in line with your upper back, either by resting on your forehead or your chin.

Go! Slowly raise both your arms and legs—keeping them straight the entire time—a few inches off the floor (or as far as you comfortably can). Hold for 3 to 4 seconds at the top, then lower your arms and legs back down. Do 8 repetitions.

The Difference Makers

- As you raise up, imagine you're trying to make your arms and legs even straighter.
- Don't overarch your back by thinking the higher you can raise your arms and legs, the better.
- Remember that it's not a race. The faster you go, the more likely you are to rely on momentum instead of your muscles. Speed can also put added stress on your lower back.
- Exhale through your mouth as you lift your arms and legs, then inhale through your nose as you lower them back to the floor.
- Finally, don't snap at the top. I want you to softly bring yourself up into position.

Why it's essential: This movement targets so many muscles that are important for overall function and performance, particularly the lower back. This is one of the easiest ways you can strengthen and protect these important core muscles. In addition, the movement engages your erector spinae muscles, the muscles alongside your spine that support it, which are crucial for back extension.

16. Alternating Arm/Leg Raise

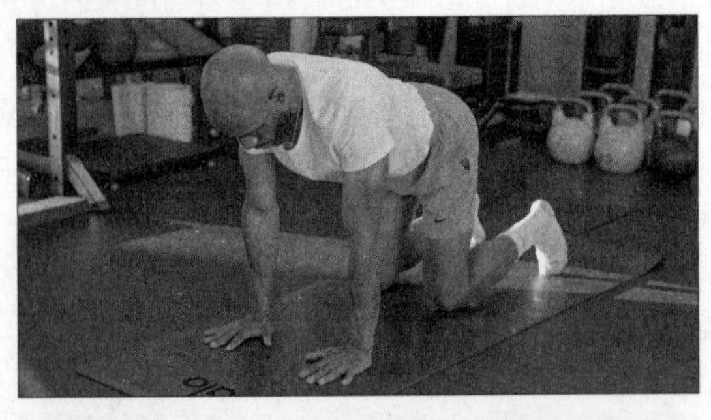

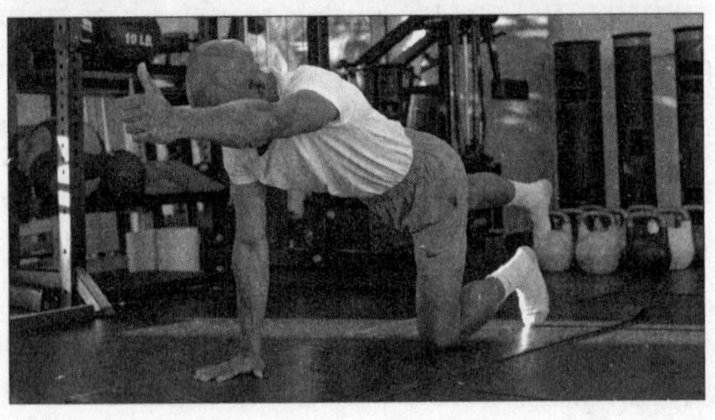

What it's working [Strengthens your core muscles (especially your lower back), erector spinae muscles, and glutes]

Ready? Get on all fours with your hands and knees spaced about hip-width apart. Your hands should be just below your shoulders and your knees should be just above your hips.

Set... Pull your stomach in and tighten your core muscles so that your torso is straight. Draw your shoulder blades in toward each other.

Go! Holding this posture, slowly extend your left arm straight out in line with your torso as you simultaneously extend your right leg straight out behind you. Hold at the top for 1 or 2 seconds, slowly reverse the motion so that you return to the Set position, then repeat the exercise, this time extending your right arm and left leg. Continue alternating back and forth for a total of 12 repetitions (6 each side).

The Difference Makers

- Don't look at where you're pointing. Your head and neck should always stay in line with your back, eyes looking toward the floor.
- Ideally, when you extend your arms, angle your hands so that your thumb points upward.

Why it's essential: This movement is not only incredibly effective at conditioning your core, but it adds a proprioceptive component that challenges your stability and trains your muscles to work synergistically to maintain balance.

17. Kneeling Hip Hinge

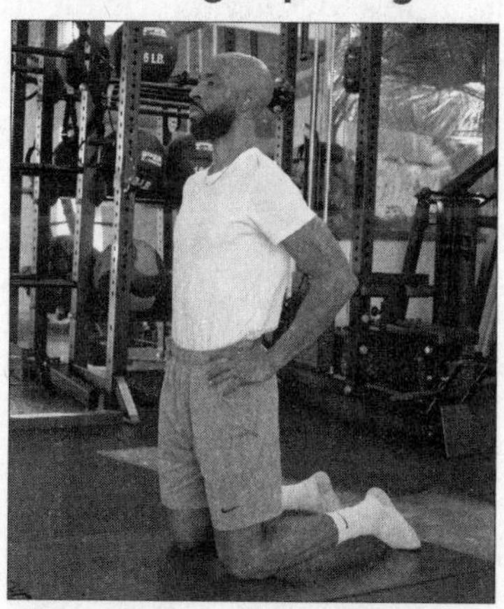

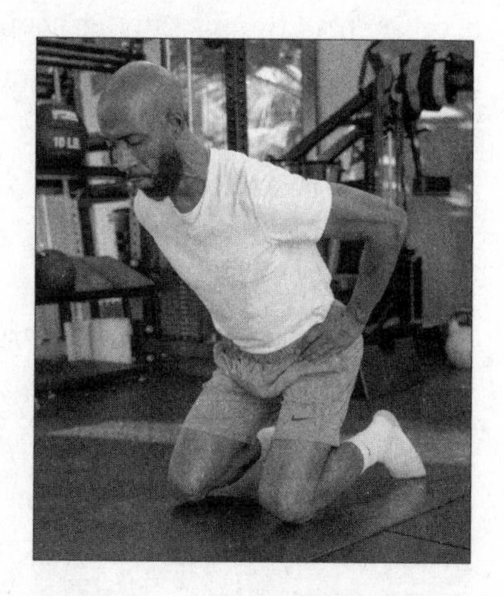

What it's working [Strengthens your hip flexors and core muscles, as well as stretches the quadriceps]

Ready? Kneel on the floor (legs bent with feet behind you). Bend your arms and place your hands gently on your hips.

Set... Face forward and position yourself so that your posture is perfect. (Your head, back, and thighs should form a straight line.)

Go! Without rounding your back, slowly tilt your hips back toward your heels as far as comfortably possible. As you go, gently bend at the waist until your torso is at a 45-degree angle from the floor. Reverse the motion until you're back in the Set position and then do 8 to 10 repetitions.

The Difference Maker

- Your torso should remain flat the entire time—don't curl it forward.

Why it's essential: Whenever you bend to lift something off the ground, not only should you bend at the knees, but you should also always bend at your hips instead of rounding your back—but that's not what most people do. Instead, they place unnecessary pressure on their lower back and discs, which can easily lead to injury. This movement is vital because in addition to strengthening your core and other muscles, it also teaches and reminds your body how and where to bend properly to avoid intrinsic pressure on your spine.

18. Single-Leg Hip Hinge

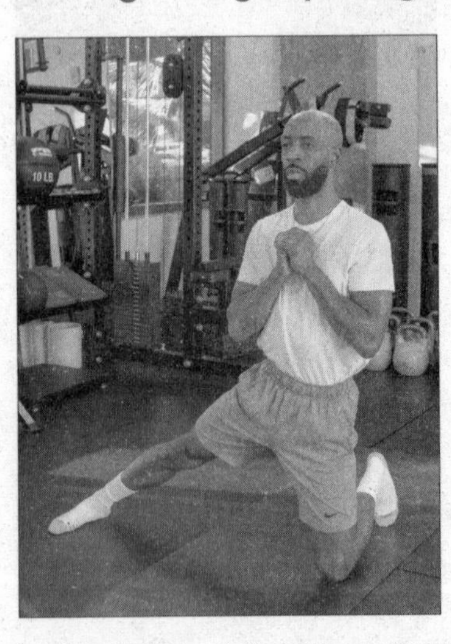

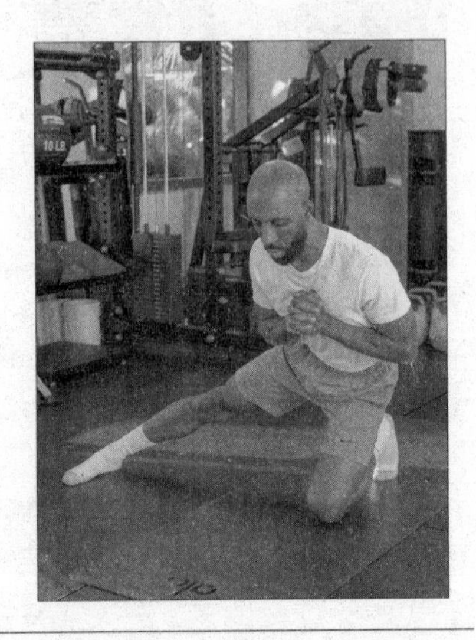

What it's working [Strengthens your core muscles, stretches the quadriceps, and stretches/strengthens the hips and groin]

Ready? Start by getting in the same position as the Kneeling Hip Hinge by kneeling on the floor, legs bent with feet behind you.

Set... Keeping your left knee on the ground, extend your right leg out to your side until it's straight. (Try to place your right foot as flat on the floor as possible for balance.) Next, bend your arms and clasp your hands together in front of your chest. Finally, face forward and position yourself so that your posture is perfect. (Your head, back, and left thigh should form a straight line.)

Go! Without rounding your back, slowly tilt your hips back toward your left heel as far as comfortably possible. As you go, gently bend at the waist until your torso is at about a 45-degree angle from the floor. Slowly reverse the movement until you're back in the Set position and do 6 to 8 repetitions.

Finish the exercise by switching positions—this time keeping your right knee on the ground and extending your left leg out to your side—for another 6 to 8 reps.

The Difference Maker

- Resist the urge to bend whichever leg is straight as you perform the exercise. You may unconsciously want to bend it for easier balance, but that only negates the stability-challenging component of the movement.

Why it's essential: Building off the exercise prior to this one in the program (the Kneeling Hip Hinge), you're still getting the same benefits, but this "next level" prime movement brings in your lower abdominal muscles, as well as works to enhance your proprioception because of the instability involved.

Better yet, it simultaneously stretches and eccentrically strengthens your groin muscles, which is a huge component toward injury prevention.

What you're doing is making your hips more flexible by opening them up with this move.

19. Ankle-Tap Downward Dog

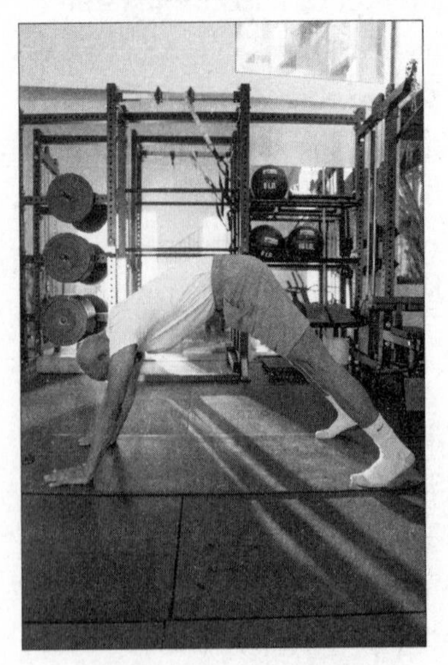

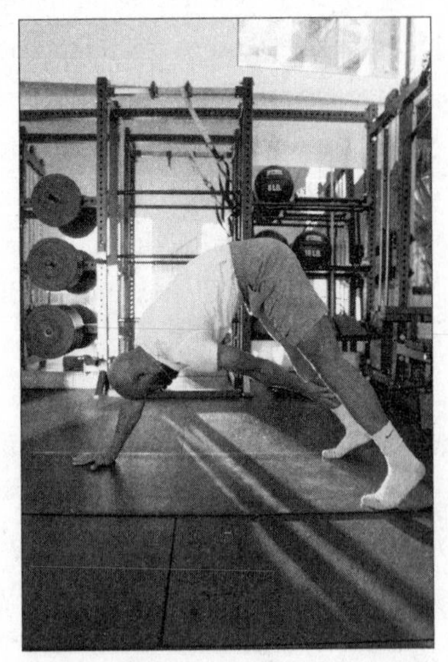

What it's working [Stretches the hamstrings, lower back, calves, and wrists, as well as strengthens the shoulders, arms, core, and wrists]

Ready? Get on all fours with your hands and knees spaced about hip-width apart. Your hands should be just below your shoulders and your knees should be just below your hips.

Set... Pull your stomach in and tighten your core muscles so that your torso is perfectly straight. Next, press through your hands as you lift your knees and raise your hips toward the ceiling. Slowly straighten your legs as you press your heels down as close as you comfortably can toward the floor—you should end up looking like an upside-down V.

Go! Holding this pose, maintain your balance as you reach back with your left hand and touch your right ankle. Return to the Set position, then repeat the exercise by reaching back with your right hand and touching your left ankle. Alternate back and forth for a total of 8 to 10 repetitions (4 to 5 each side).

The Difference Maker

- Don't let the movement cause you to break form, especially with your upper body—your arms, head, and torso should form a straight line and stay that way.

Why it's essential: This modification on a classic yoga position—which I call a "downward dog hamstring posterior chain active mobility stretch" (try saying *that* five times fast)—not only conditions your posterior chain muscles, but also helps improve rotation mobility of the spine. That combination targets many of the muscle groups that most people typically pull or strain when they lack flexibility in these areas.

20. Spider-Man Stretch

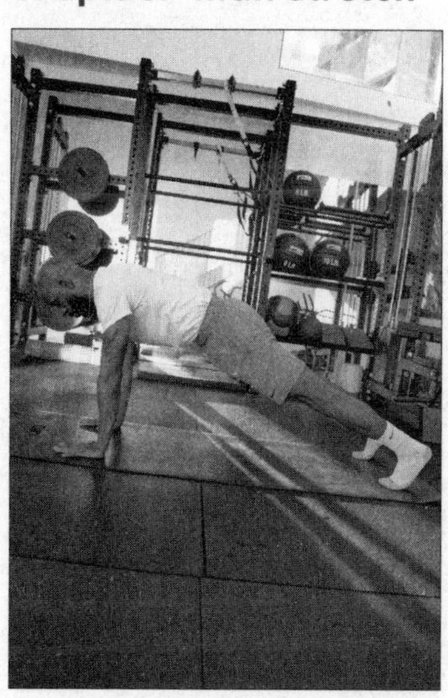

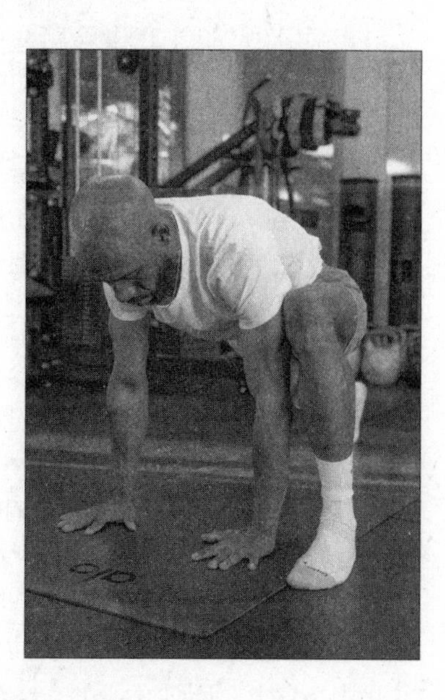

What it's working [Loosens and opens up the hips, stretching both your adductors and hamstrings]

Ready? Get in a classic push-up position with your hands flat on the floor (shoulder-width apart), arms straight, and your legs straight behind you with your weight on your toes (or the tops of the balls of your feet).

Set... Pull in your stomach and contract your core muscles.

Go! Keeping your hands flat on the floor, lift your left foot and step forward with your left leg. Plant your left foot just outside of your left hand, then shift your hips forward as far as you comfortably can. Return to the Set position, then repeat the stretch, this time stepping forward with your right leg and planting your right foot just outside of your right hand. Alternate back and forth for a total of 8 to 10 repetitions (4 to 5 each side).

The Difference Makers

- Don't touch just your heel to the floor each time you step. Try to plant your foot as flat as possible every time.
- Everyone is different when it comes to their hip mobility, so your foot may not completely reach your hand—and that's fine. However, don't bring your feet too close to your rib cage. That can put unnecessary pressure on your lower back.
- Move at your own pace, but if you do it too fast, there's a risk of pinching your back a little.

Why it's essential: This stretch easily transfers over into daily life. It promotes hip mobility and flexion, so the more you practice it, the more you're likely to lift using your legs as opposed to your back.

The Stand-to-Command Finale

It's time to get back on your feet and finish strong with these final seven movements. But listen . . . just because you're almost finished doesn't mean you can coast through this final portion. Strive to give these last few the same amount of focus and energy that you did at the start!

21. Standing Pelvic Tilt

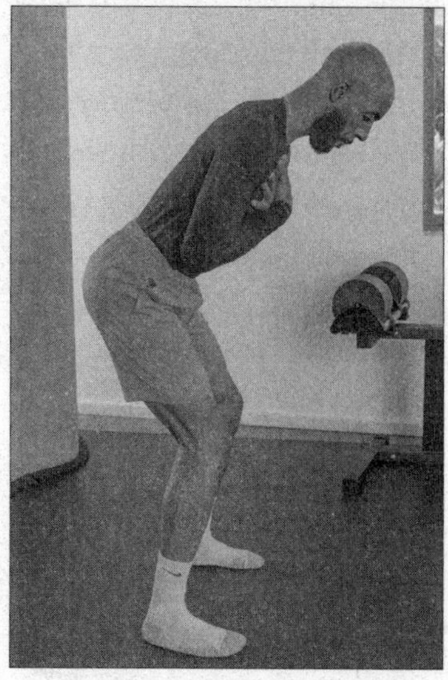

What it's working [Loosens the hips, stretches the erector spine and hamstrings (as well as eccentrically strengthens your hams), and promotes spinal mobility]

Ready? Stand straight with your feet shoulder-width apart, knees slightly bent. Cross your arms over your chest and place your hands on your shoulders.

Set . . . From the waist, lean forward slightly (just an inch or two) as if you were standing over your golf ball on the tee. Pull in your stomach and tighten your midsection to engage your core muscles.

Go! Holding this position, slowly tilt your hips forward and hold for a second. Next, slowly tilt your hips backward and hold for another second. (Going back and forth counts as 1 repetition.) Continue to tilt your hips back and forth for a total of 8 to 10 repetitions.

The Difference Maker

- The only movement should be your hips. If anything else is bending or rocking back and forth, you're not focusing on your form and/or you're going too fast.

Why it's essential: This might be the easiest exercise in this program—and yet it's absolutely essential in creating both spinal awareness and mobility within the lumbar spine.

So many people throw out their backs—even when lifting the lightest amounts of weight—often because their bodies are too rigid. This easy-to-do move is a game-changer in terms of minimizing injury because it teaches you to engage your core while moving your hips simultaneously, which grants you more flexibility in the lumbar region. It also gives you an awareness of your lower back and how to move it efficiently.

22. Thoracic Spine Rotation

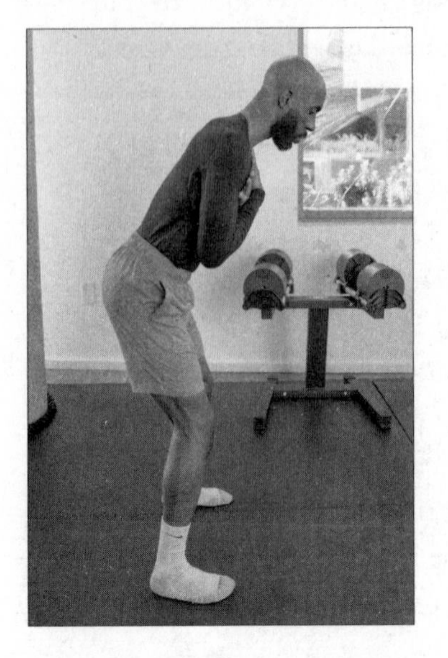

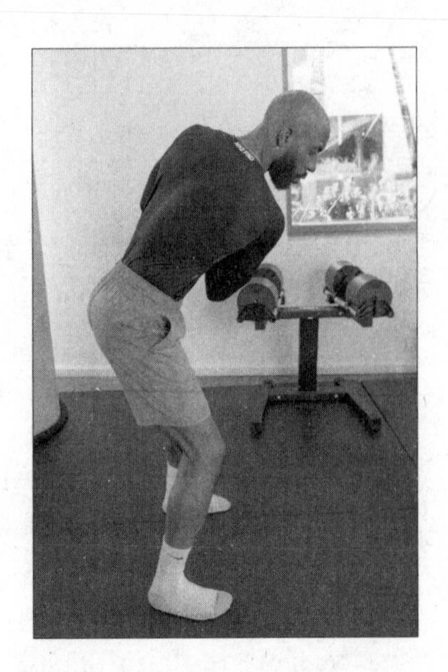

What it's working [Isolates and loosens up the thoracic spine for increased mobility and control within the upper and midback]

Ready? For this move, you'll get into the same position as the Standing Pelvic Tilt. Stand straight with your feet shoulder-width apart, knees slightly bent. Cross your arms over your chest and place your hands on your shoulders.

Set... From the waist, lean forward slightly (just an inch or two) as if you were angling yourself to use a golf club. Pull in your stomach and tighten your midsection to engage your core muscles.

Go! Holding this position, rotate your shoulders to the left as far as you comfortably can, then rotate your shoulders to the right as far as you comfortably can. (That's 1 repetition.) Continue rotating from left to right for a total of 10 repetitions.

The Difference Makers

- Only your upper back should move—your head and neck should stay straight, and your lower back and legs should remain locked and as stiff as a board. If you're bending any of the above (especially your knees), it means you're trying to get a greater range of motion, but all you're doing is minimizing the effectiveness of the movement.
- Imagine your goal is to position your shoulder just below your chin, but don't force it. If you're not quite that flexible yet, it will come with time.

Why it's essential: This rotational activation stretch goes together with the Standing Pelvic Tilt to train your body to move in a way that protects your lumbar spine, preventing you from suffering from slipped discs and lower back pain.

As you rotate your shoulders, you're mobilizing your thoracic spine, the section that begins at the base of your neck and stops at the bottom of your rib cage. These twelve discs (T1 through T12) are the ones that decide your spine's range of motion, so as you improve mobility in this area, you're decreasing the risk of injury to your spine and lower back.

23. Single-Leg Balance Oscillation

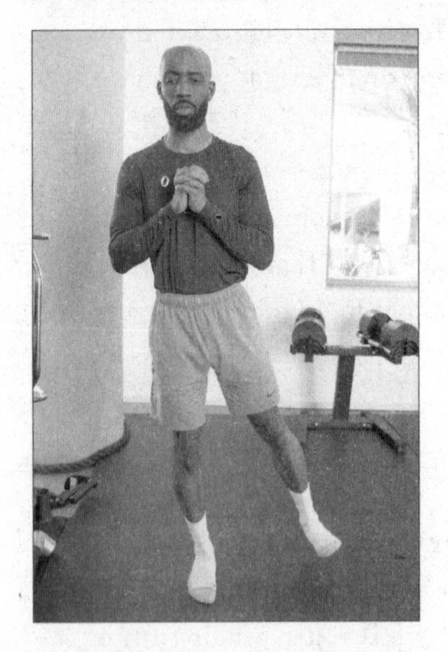

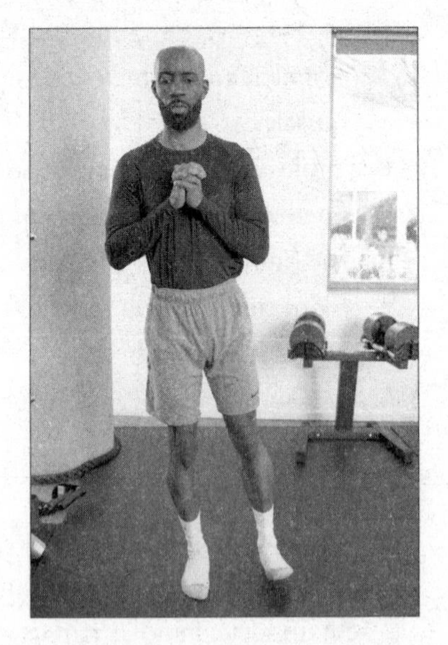

What it's working [Conditions your lower core muscles, as well as your hips, lower back, glutes, groin, and adductors]

Ready? Stand straight with your hands clasped together in front of your chest, facing forward with your chin up.

Set... Raise your left foot just off the floor so that your left leg is slightly extended out to the side. Contract your midsection so that your core is tight.

Go! Holding this posture, move your left leg in and out from side to side as quickly as you can without shifting yourself off-balance. (Going left then right counts as 1 repetition.) Do 25 repetitions with each leg.

The Difference Makers

- Nothing should be moving except your leg. If you're doing it right, your core and the glute muscles on your stationary leg will be on fire.

- Keep your eyes forward and resist the urge to look down—don't worry, your foot's not going anywhere.

Why it's essential: Training the lower core and the adductors/groin is something commonly neglected, which is why so many people suffer strains in these areas, even when they stretch often and try to be careful. But in addition to conditioning these muscle groups, this simple yet effective movement also adds a neural component by challenging your proprioceptive muscles. Your body is constantly having to maintain its balance as you perform the movement, so you're teaching it to be reactive in a way that's beneficial in sports, activities, and everyday life.

24. Sumo Lateral Squat

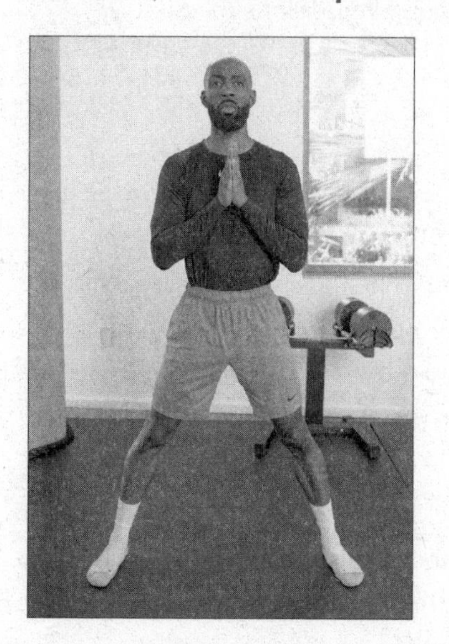

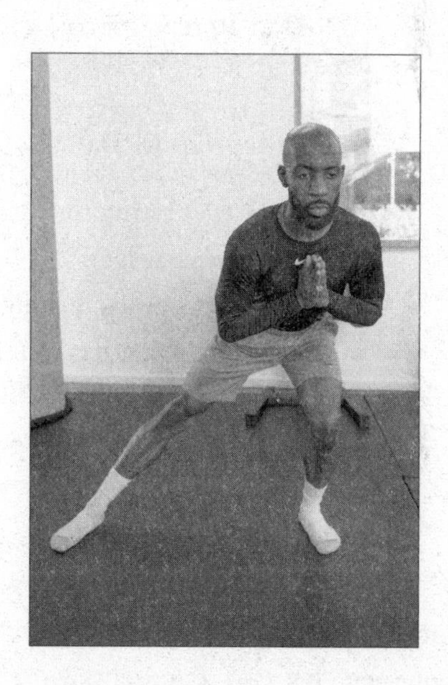

What it's working [Strengthens the glutes, quadriceps, hamstrings, calves, and core muscles]

Ready? Stand straight with your feet wider than shoulder-width apart pointing slightly out to the sides. Put your hands together—palms flat against each other as if you're praying—directly in front of you.

Set... Contract your abdominals so that your core muscles are engaged. Keep your head and neck in line with your back and face forward.

Go! Lower your body by bending your left knee only—your right leg will remain straight—until your left thigh is almost parallel to the floor. Your head and torso should remain upright and facing forward—not angled toward your bent leg. Hold this position for 1 or 2 seconds, push yourself back up into the Set position, and repeat—but this time, bend your right knee only and keep your left leg straight until your right thigh is almost parallel to the floor. Do 8 to 10 repetitions total (4 or 5 repetitions for each leg).

The Difference Makers

- Keep your eyes facing forward the entire time. Resist the urge to look down at your legs.
- As odd as this sounds, I want you to imagine that you're about to sit on a chair that has room for only one glute—the glute of whichever leg is bending. When you use this trick, it helps you isolate that singular muscle group, rather than relying upon both glutes.

Why it's essential: What I love about this move is how it improves unilateral muscular balance by teaching the body to support itself on one leg. It's also an essential exercise for improving stability in your knees and ankles, in addition to conditioning your legs in a way that protects your knees from injury. Another benefit is that it's a dynamic stretch that simultaneously improves your range of motion and flexibility as it strengthens your muscles.

25. Split-Stance Isometric Wall Squat

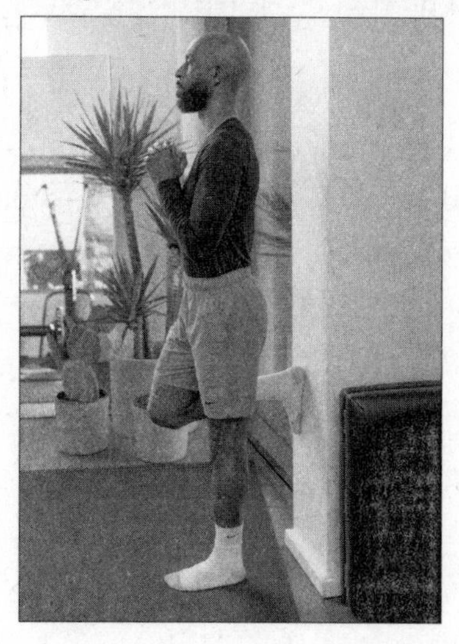

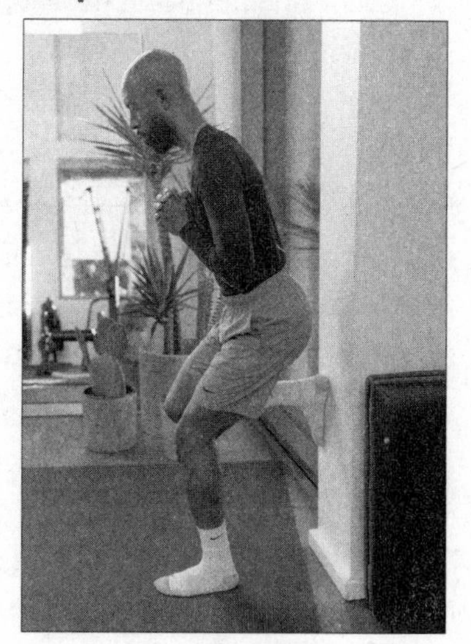

What it's working [Strengthens the glutes, quadriceps, and core muscles]

Ready? Find a sturdy wall and stand at least 12 inches away from it. Bend your right leg and place your right foot flat on the wall. Bring your hands up in front of your chest and make a pair of fists.

Set... Make sure that you're standing with perfect posture. Your chin should be up, and your core should be engaged.

Go! Slowly bend your left leg and squat down as far as you comfortably can. Hold this position for 20 seconds, then repeat the move—but this time place your left foot on the wall and squat using your right leg.

The Difference Makers

- The deeper you can go down, the better—but stop once the thigh of your working leg is parallel to the floor.
- Some consider this move more demanding than others (depending on the length of their legs), so to keep your mind off

your muscles being worked, focus on your breathing instead of the burn.

Why it's essential: This weightless variation of a bodyweight squat lets you isometrically load your quadriceps one leg at a time. To do this exercise, all the tendons and muscles that support your knee must fire, strengthening each knee individually with minimal equipment and minimal load (so it's an incredibly safe way to condition them).

26. Single-Leg Romanian Deadlift (RDL)

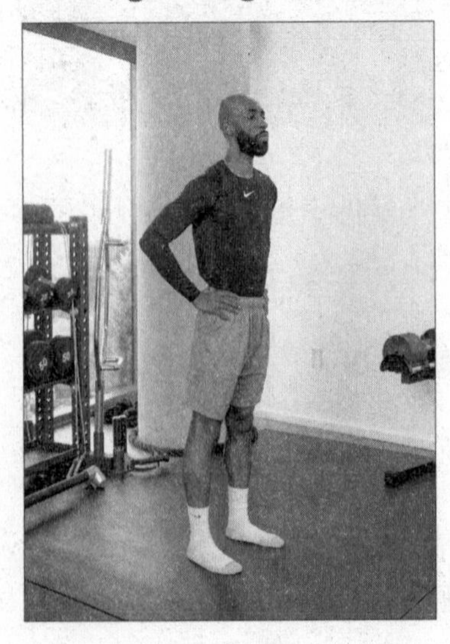

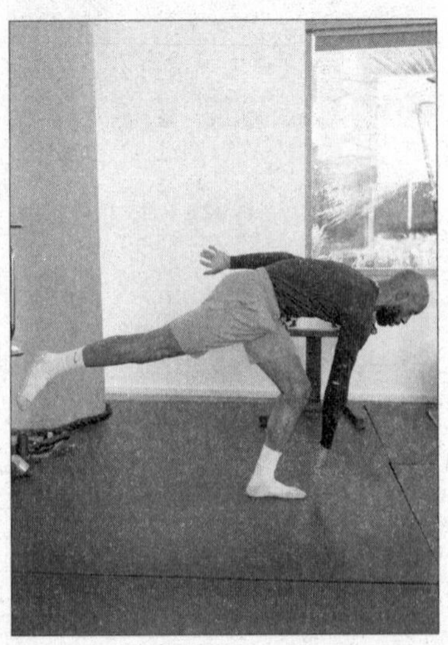

What it's working [Strengthens your hamstrings, glutes, erector spinae, calves, and core—basically all your posterior chain muscles]

Ready? Stand with your feet roughly shoulder-width apart and your hands on your hips. Your knees should be unlocked.
Set . . . Contract your core muscles as you lift your right foot up behind you about an inch off the floor—you should be balancing on your left foot.
Go! Keeping your core engaged, push your hips back and bend at the waist to lower your torso toward the floor. Your right leg

should simultaneously extend behind you. Stop when your torso is almost parallel to the floor (or if you notice tightness in your hamstrings and glutes), then squeeze your glutes to reverse the motion until you're back in the Set position.

Repeat the exercise balancing on your left leg for 6 to 10 repetitions, then switch positions to work the opposite leg (this time, balancing on your right foot and extending your left leg backward).

The Difference Maker

- Don't just let your torso drop. As you lower yourself down, control the pace and don't let gravity do the work.

Why it's essential: Single-leg Romanian deadlifts not only recruit and strengthen all your posterior chain muscles, but this dynamic hinge movement also improves mobility (especially in the hamstrings) and teaches proper functioning of the hips, in addition to helping you develop better single-leg stability.

27. Rocket Ship

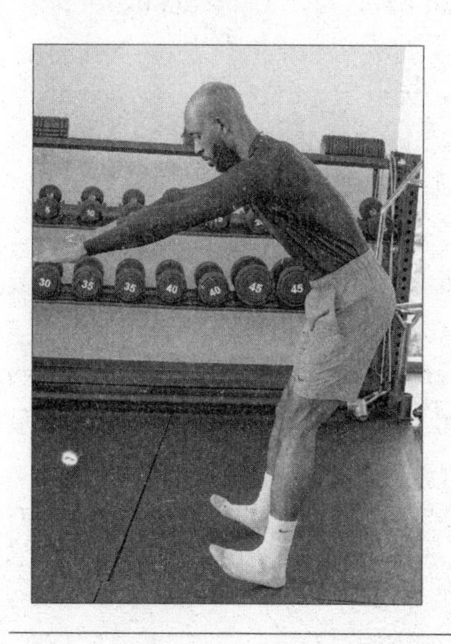

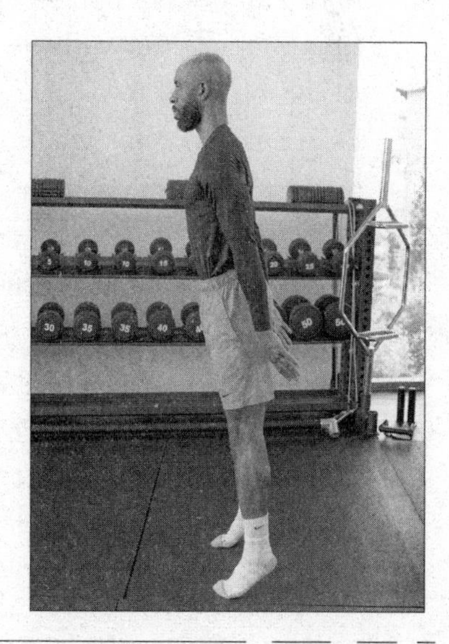

What it's working: [Strengthens your core muscles, quadriceps, hamstrings, glutes, and calves]

Ready? Stand straight with your feet slightly wider than shoulder-width apart and your arms straight down at your sides. Your legs should be straight with your knees unlocked.

Set... First, engage your core by tightening your abdominals. Then slowly push your butt back as you extend your arms in front of you, palms down. Finally, slowly raise your toes so that you're balancing on your heels. (Note: It may take you a couple seconds—or even a couple tries—to get into this starting position, but that's okay. Your form will get better over time.)

Go! Once you're balanced, shift your hips forward and stand up on your toes, letting your arms swing behind you. Hold at the top for 2 or 3 seconds, then reverse the motion back into the Set position and repeat 8 to 10 times.

The Difference Makers

- Don't just pop onto your toes. Instead, you should be rolling from your heels to your toes, then reversing the motion by rolling from your toes to your heels.
- At the top of the movement, raise your chest up as far as you can.
- Each time you come back down, tilt your hips back as if you're about to sit on a chair.

Why it's essential: I like to end with this move for two reasons. First, it puts everything together. The program starts with your feet and finishes with your feet, but this movement forces you to integrate what you've worked on in the rest of the program, activating your entire foundation from the hips down.

Second, I find it inspiring. During those last few repetitions, your ankles might be shaking, and your abs may feel like they're on fire—but once you get through it, you'll be ready to attack the day. The movement itself looks like you're confidently charging forward, like a skier sailing off a ramp or a superhero flying from a building—fearless and prepared. You got this, and now, because of the time you just invested in yourself, so does your body.

THAT'S IT—YOU'RE DONE!

Everything is engaged and stabilized, particularly your core and posture. Your physical and mental awareness have been jump-started, and you should immediately feel more energized, confident, flexible, body aware—and, especially, more functional.

You're not just going through the motions today—you *own* your motions. Every single movement you make from this point forward will have more power, speed, and coordination, no matter which direction your body moves or what activity you decide to take on.

Now go. Get your kids ready for school. Hit that board meeting. Let's attack the day!

For supplementary material from Mike Mancias, please visit:

CHAPTER 9

Break It Down

Let's get real here.

Why did you pick up this book? You're reading it because you're looking for something more from your life. Whether it's finally pulling off the healthier lifestyle you've never been able to achieve, augmenting your performance in your sport of choice, or just feeling as young as possible for as long as possible, you're looking for something more from yourself. But whatever you've been doing up until now, you've just been going through the motions and getting by.

If you're not completely satisfied or happy with the direction your body has traveled up until this point—how it looks, how it feels, and how it performs—the only way to change that direction is to be brutally honest each and every time you execute my mobility regimen. You owe it to yourself to take inventory of the effort you put into it, whether this is your first time doing my program or your thousandth. You owe it to yourself to determine how well you were able to follow through with it, as well as to assess how it made you feel—and function—for the rest of the day.

You see, a lot of people just go through the motions when it comes to exercise, do what they have to do, and consider themselves a success if they managed to do something active that day. But just because you finished my mobility regimen doesn't necessarily mean you broke ground on constructing a better body. Your body is an incredible adaptive machine, capable of transforming into something beyond what you ever thought you were even capable of becoming. But it's also stubborn; it only changes when it feels that it must. Go through the motions, just so you can say that you exercised, and your body will know. That type of "phoning it in" fitness is why most people never evolve into what they were meant to become. That's why I always say to my clients that once the hard work is done, that's when the actual work starts—and the real change begins.

This chapter is all about taking a serious look at what went right and what went wrong. Were there distractions that kept you from focusing on proper form? A situation that forced you to rush through the regimen instead of taking time with it? Don't worry if you're not sure right now, because you soon will be. It's time to pull apart what you *really* did—to look for what could've silently sabotaged your success (so we can put an end to it) and/or figure out what pushed you to be your best (so we can keep that mojo coming).

If you ran into problems with any of the twenty-seven movements—either because certain ones were too difficult or too easy—the next chapter will show you how to modify each move individually to match your current fitness level. But for now, I want you to think about the following three specific areas of interest.

1. How Do You Feel Now Compared to Then?

It's time to grab that "body baseline"—the five questions I asked you to answer about yourself prior to the routine—to see if anything's changed.

1. **Do you feel sore in any of these areas (circle all that apply)?**
   Feet. Ankles. Calves/Achilles. Hamstrings. Quadriceps. Hips. Midsection. Lower Back. Upper Back. Shoulders. Arms. Neck.
2. **Do you feel tight/stiff in any of these areas (circle all that apply)?**
   Feet. Ankles. Calves/Achilles. Hamstrings. Quadriceps. Hips. Midsection. Lower Back. Upper Back. Shoulders. Arms. Neck.

3. **Do you feel weak in any of these areas (circle all that apply)?**
   Feet. Ankles. Calves/Achilles. Hamstrings. Quadriceps. Hips. Midsection. Lower Back. Upper Back. Shoulders. Arms. Neck.

4. **Where would you rank your energy level?**
   (1 being the least alert; 10 being the most alert):
   1 2 3 4 5 6 7 8 9 10

5. **Where would you rank your motivation?**
   (1 being "just phoning it in"; 10 being "ready to crush this"):
   1 2 3 4 5 6 7 8 9 10

Now, let me say this right off the bat: Don't expect every area to notice an improvement—even though that's certainly possible, depending on the day. Instead, just look for any differences. Some may be undeniable, others subtle, while a few might even be undetectable at first until you go about your day and notice an improvement.

Do not skip this step. It literally takes two minutes of your time, and it might be the most important two minutes of your day. One of the biggest reasons people have a hard time staying consistent with a routine is that their expectations are tied to long-term goals: hitting a specific number on the scale, lifting a certain amount of weight a certain number of times, shaving seconds off their 5K personal record. They follow a program that may require months to reach their goals. But because they're not seeing instant results, it's hard for them to stay the course.

The reason I insist on doing this with clients is to get them to really pay attention to what's happening with their body immediately afterward, something very few people bother to do after working out. Maybe you think that's not the case—and I get it. If you're normally active, I'm sure that after a workout you're already aware of the obvious. Maybe you noticed how it kicked your ass or how sore your muscles felt afterward, but that type of surface understanding can only take you so far if you're shooting for consistency.

Revisiting your body baseline immediately after performing my routine forces you to look at every portion of your body from top to bottom to see if it feels less sore, less stiff, or less weak. It gets you to acknowledge that you have more energy, even though technically you should feel slightly tired because, after all, you just completed a workout.

Finally, it tracks whether you're walking away from the routine feeling more or less motivated than when you started. Quickly re-examining the five "body baseline" factors gives you that instant gratification that what you're *hoping* to accomplish *is* being accomplished, and that will keep you coming back tomorrow and every tomorrow after that.

2. What Took It to the Next Level?

Something caused you to push yourself harder, feel more accomplished, or look forward to the program this time around—so what was it exactly? Sometimes it's a combination of factors, while other times it might just be one. Whatever it was for you today—when doing my mobility program or during any physical activity that challenged your body—if you want to channel that feeling again, then you need to piece together what caused it in the first place.

Atmosphere: Chances are, the spot you've chosen to do my routine—whether it's at home or in the gym—is most likely where you'll do it tomorrow and the next day after that. So if there was something about that environment that made it easier for you to complete the program—anything that you believe might have made you more motivated, even just a little bit—then acknowledge it.

For example, was it the lighting, the time of day, or the weather? Did you look at a picture of someone you care about? Hear a particular song playing in the background? Smell coffee from the kitchen or the flowers from the garden? Were you enjoying the convenience of being able to do it from home? I don't want you to think too hard about it, but reflect for a moment and try to connect with at least one thing that added to the experience. That way, you can take extra steps to keep it in place for next time or try to re-create it someplace else when traveling or anytime you find yourself out of your natural element.

Outside inspiration: Motivation can come from any direction. It could be praise from others, wanting to be healthier for your family, something that you heard or read, or even remembering you need to be in better shape for a particular event. I don't know what might have left you more determined to get the most from a workout this time around, so what was it?

Were you recognized and given credit for something at work? Was it that article about the positive effects of exercise you happened to scroll upon on your phone, or some mantra you saw on a poster? Was it something someone you admire said or did? Did you notice you were able to do something physically with less effort—or maybe for the first time—because of the program? Is there an upcoming situation you want to be sure you're prepared for, such as a vacation, a class reunion, or a father-son event at school?

Organization: Sometimes, feeling like you have all your sh*t together in one area of your life can make other areas more manageable. This program is designed not to require too much planning or thinking, but it still takes effort, and if getting a better handle on the rest of your day took some of the pressure off doing my routine, then you must validate that.

Acceptance: As I mentioned earlier in this chapter, it's important to recognize the importance of what you're doing and how it's positively affecting your life *in the moment*. Many people just go through the motions and do what they're told. They run through every exercise or stretch as if it's Twister, putting their arms and legs wherever the spinner lands and a workout routine tells them to. They never really spend a second thinking about *why* they're moving a certain way. But when you give each movement its due by recognizing it—when you're present and truly thinking about how your body is benefiting from each action as you're doing it—that can add fuel into your tank when you need it most.

3. What Stood in the Way of Success?

First, put any guilt aside if, for some reason, you didn't put in as much effort into the routine as you could have. You're far from alone. All my clients face obstacles that sometimes keep them from being 100 percent in the zone every single session, and that's okay. Something is always better than nothing. However, drilling down on what could be preventing you from giving it your all, especially if it's something that's consistently happening, is necessary. If you don't get to the bottom of what is holding you back, you'll never reach the top. That's why I ask my clients to think about what stood in their way so they can put together a better approach to prevent those issues from happening the next time.

Impatience: Did you rush through the workout? Even if you're not sure, there's an easy way to tell: Time yourself from the moment you start until the moment you finish. On average, the entire routine as prescribed should take you approximately twenty minutes or so (which accounts for how long it takes on average to get into each position). If your number falls below that time frame—and nothing else had distracted you—then chances are, you did certain movements for less time or fewer repetitions than recommended.

Is that you? If that's the case, ask yourself, "Why did I shave off those seconds?" If you had to get something done or be someplace, I get it—that's life. But if cutting those corners is happening more frequently than not, then consider the fact that putting in 90 percent of the effort means getting back 90 percent of the results if you're lucky. Are those few minutes you're saving worth missing out on the other 10 percent? I think you know the answer to that.

And consider this: The more you complete the program, the more familiar you'll become with it—and the quicker it will go. Whether you're a beginner or advanced, I'm fully expecting you to take a little longer to get into each move and to defer to the book to make sure that you're doing it right. All those starts and stops add up to a slightly longer workout, but it's extra time that's helping you double-check what you're doing, and that's important. Don't worry . . . it doesn't take long to master every movement.

Priorities: I've never met anyone—no matter their level of professional success—who didn't believe they were busy. From athletes and entertainers to blue-collar and white-collar workers, from high schoolers to house moms—we all have stuff going on because that's how life works.

Is that you? Then ask yourself, "Why is that thing that kept me from giving it my all with the program so important to me?" Obviously, there will always be certain pressing matters that have to be placed on top of the to-do list, but if you're noticing it's becoming a frequent issue that's getting in your way, then consider this: Does it give you back something of equal benefit? If not, then don't let it get in your way. If it's important, then is it something you could schedule at a different time that doesn't interfere with the routine, and if not, can you find a better time to do the routine, so they never conflict with each other?

But here's the real kicker: *If you had stuck with the program as prescribed . . . is it possible you could have been even "more" effective/successful with whatever that priority was?* For example, maybe you phoned it in because you had to help a friend move or coach your daughter's soccer team. If it was something physical you had to do, it's a given that you would've been able to carry out that task more effectively *if* you had stuck with the program. And even if it wasn't anything physical, would approaching that priority with more confidence have helped you?

Personal: It's okay to let your mind wander doing some of the movements in my mobility program, so long as it's not preventing you from focusing on them and keeping perfect form. However, if you're going through something (whether at work, home, or elsewhere) that's overwhelming you to the point that you can't concentrate and give the routine 100 percent effort, that's a problem to address.

Is that you? Because everyone is different, I can't predict what personal issues you might pull into your workout, but I do know this: Doing a quick assessment to see if what's bothering you is something that matters more than doing the mobility workout is easy enough to do. All it takes is looking at what took up real estate in your brain that day and answering the following:

Drama or dire? In other words, is what's bothering you something that others would shake their head at, or would they be genuinely concerned? For the most part, we know the difference between what's important and what deserves nothing more than an eye roll.

Pressing or postponable? Whatever that catastrophe was that you couldn't shake, was it something that needed to be handled ASAP—or could it have waited at least another thirty minutes until you were finished?

Finally, I've had some clients not be able to focus because exercising when they were going through a crisis felt selfish to them, especially if what was on their minds was someone else and problems they might be going through. That makes perfect sense, but if that's you, realize that by spending a few minutes each day taking care of yourself, you'll be putting yourself in a better position to take care of others. It's not selfish to allow a few moments to improve yourself so that nothing stands in your way to be there for them when they need you.

Pride: What I'm asking of you is no different from what I ask of any of my clients, many of whom are professional athletes. But sometimes I've watched people I've worked with go from 100 to 0 mph just because they made a mistake midway through. Maybe they found themselves a little weaker or tighter that morning in a specific movement, or maybe they couldn't hold a certain pose or stretch quite as far as they usually do. Then they spend the rest of the workout beating themselves up over it.

Is that you? If so, know this: So long as you're staying true to my mobility program and doing all twenty-seven movements, no one is judging you for how well you're doing them. If I was standing in front of you, I would correct your form if you were doing something incorrectly and encourage you to work to your potential, but judging somebody for what they're able or unable to do isn't who I am—and not who I want you to be. I don't expect perfection, but I do expect persistence. So if your self-esteem is taking the steam out of your effort, put a stop to it right now. Remember what I said at the beginning of this book: You may lose the battle with certain movements on certain days, but by sticking it out and giving it your best, you will never fail.

Pain: We all have a different threshold for pain, but the movements in my program shouldn't hurt—unless you're performing them incorrectly, overdoing it, or have other issues going on with you physically. When it comes to mobility and core strength, every move in the program is a high-caliber movement that delivers results while minimizing the risk of injury.

That's why it's important to recognize the difference between actual pain versus discomfort/soreness, as I mentioned earlier in the book. If before starting this program you've lived more of a sedentary lifestyle, then you can expect some muscle soreness to occur and last for at least a few weeks as your body becomes more acclimated with the program. Remember, you're asking your body to do movements it hasn't done in a while (or perhaps ever). Soreness in your joints, tendons, and muscles is a natural but temporary side effect that means the program is working—so keep at it!

Is that you? Obviously if you ever feel a pop, snap, or strain when performing any movement, then immediately back off and have it checked out because there's a different issue there you need to address. Otherwise, listen to your body. Is it a pain that recently started or one that you've had for a while and a certain movement within the program is calling attention to it? Is it possible that other activities you're doing in addition to the program—working out, participating in sports, doing housework, having a physical job, etc.—could be the culprit for the stress you're feeling on that particular area?

Like I said, none of the twenty-seven movements should hurt unless you're doing them wrong—in fact, they're meant to minimize your everyday aches and pains—so stick with the regimen and try pulling back on extracurricular activities that could be pushing certain portions of your body too hard and too often. If after a week you still feel discomfort or pain from a particular movement, there could be an underlying issue you may want to bring to the attention of your healthcare provider.

Pooped: Even though my routine challenges you in different ways in terms of stability, stamina, and strength, it's not an exhausting workout. In fact, when you do it right, you'll feel more energized and ready to take on the world afterward. So if you're too tired at any point during my routine, it shouldn't be because it's too much to handle. The problem most likely is tied to something else you're doing.

Is that you? There are a variety of reasons you could be fizzling out, some of which should correct themselves as you adopt and follow through with the other portions of the book (Eat and Mend):

You might be overtraining. Exercise, sports, and any activity that places a physical demand on your body—when done too much—can lead to overtraining, so if you're performing additional activities on top of my program, it could be overtaxing your muscles and central nervous system. In the Mend section, I'll show you an easy way to check for that, and what you can do about it.

You might be hungry. First off, you shouldn't be. Even though my preference is to perform my mobility routine first thing in the morning, as I mentioned earlier in the book, having something small to eat immediately after waking up keeps your body from breaking down hard-earned lean muscle tissue for energy, so your belly should already be satisfied. However, if you're not the type to eat before exercise, start small and consider having a piece of fruit, such as a banana or a handful of berries. Or you can split up your breakfast and have a small portion of it before you start (then finish the rest of it afterward). Finally, you could sip on a shake during some of the less-intense movements if that's more convenient for you. What I don't want is for you to have a full stomach prior to or during the routine, since that can leave you bloated and could impact both your mobility and comfort level preforming certain movements.

You might be dehydrated. In the Eat portion of the book, I discussed the importance of hydration and precisely how I want you to drink throughout the day—so be honest with yourself. Were your hydration levels where they should've been prior to taking on the routine that day? If not—or you can't even remember how much you had to drink beforehand—chances are that being slightly dehydrated could've affected your energy.

You might be sleep-deprived. If you're not guilty of anything I've just mentioned (and you're not sick, potentially coming down with something, or have some other underlying health issue that could be zapping your energy), lack of sleep—or not enough *deep* sleep—is most likely the cause. In the Mend section later in the book, I'll discuss the importance of sleep and how you can achieve not just a better night's rest but the best rest possible.

CHAPTER 10

Rebuild It Better

My mobility regimen is designed so that you can do it anywhere. The twenty-seven movements are also easily adaptable, allowing you to effortlessly modify them to make each either more accessible or more complex, depending on where you are at in your fitness journey.

That said, what I want you to keep in mind is that although this chapter offers ways to intensify the regimen, that doesn't mean I want you to immediately rush to do so. Some of the movements require time to take full effect, but the longer you use them, the more they'll collectively make a difference in your mobility. Follow the program as prescribed for at least two or three weeks before considering ways to intensify any of the movements. However, if a particular exercise is giving you problems right away, then this section should be utilized immediately.

How to Modify the Mobility Movements

Rebuilding each of the twenty-seven movements—either to make them slightly easier until you master them or to accentuate them so that you see more results—isn't rocket science. In most cases, it just takes:

playing with the numbers (by raising either the repetitions or the seconds);
adding more weight (by incorporating weights into the movement);

altering the tempo (by doing a movement either slower or faster);

or **changing the surface you're standing on to affect your stability** (by using a WAFF balance disc or anything that challenges your balance and central nervous system).

That said, the following section will show you how to tweak each of the twenty-seven movements to match your current abilities.

The Tools That Intensify!

To augment certain movements, you'll need to invest in a couple specific—but inexpensive—pieces of equipment that help create a more unstable surface. No matter which one you use, each of these add-ons will allow you to recruit even more muscle fibers throughout your glutes, core, and other muscle groups to assist stabilizing you:

Two foam rollers (short and long): These cylindrical tubes come in all shapes and sizes but having just two of them (one that's less than 12 inches long, as well as a long one around 36 inches long) will run you only about 20 dollars each.

An inflatable balance disc: Also sometimes referred to as a "wobble cushion," it's an air-filled disc you can also find for around 20 dollars. Tip: Investing in two will give you more options when you become more advanced. My personal preference above all others is the WAFF inflatable disc balance cushion. I found this model to be the most portable and durable on the market, giving you the flexibility to take it anywhere (making it excuse-proof) without having to worry about it deflating on you when you're on the road.

A stability ball: These oversized inflatable balls leave your body little choice but to engage your core muscles to stay balanced on them, whether you use them to sit, rest your feet on, or hold on to.

[Note: When traveling, you could also use a small pillow or a rolled-up towel in place of these pieces of equipment wherever I'm suggesting using them. Pillows and towels won't create as unstable a surface, but at least you'll have options when you don't have access to these other items.]

1. Plantar Fascia Stretch

Make it more manageable by:

- **Trying a different tool.** You can use any type of ball, so feel free to experiment if a tennis ball feels too soft (two choices a lot of athletes like to use include a lacrosse ball or even a golf ball). You can also try a rolling pin or a frozen bottle of water to loosen up your plantar fascia—it's all about what feels better for your feet.

Elevate the intensity by:

- **Gripping the ball.** Each time the ball reaches the front of your foot, grab it with your toes and squeeze it for a second, then release.
- **Doing a heel pump.** Every time the ball reaches the back of your foot, keep the ball tucked underneath your heel and gently push up and down a few times.

2. Standing Wall Stretch

Make it more manageable by:

- **Adjusting your stance.** If your calf muscles and Achilles tendon are so tight that dropping your heel down to the floor is impossible, try bringing your back leg an inch or two closer to the wall.

Elevate the intensity by:

- **Holding the movement a little longer.** Each time you bend your forward leg and feel the stretch in your back leg, pause for a few seconds.
- **Adding some oscillation.** Instead of keeping your back foot on the ground the entire time, try this after every repetition:

Immediately raise the knee of your back leg up in front of you until your upper thigh is parallel to the floor, then reverse the movement to get back into the Set position.

3. Standing Hamstring and Nerve Floss Stretch

Make it more manageable by:

- **Holding on to something.** Ideally, I want both of your arms moving at the same time. But if it's impossible for you to do the move without using a nearby chair, table, or anything sturdy to support yourself with one arm, that's fine until you get the hang of things.

Elevate the intensity by:

- **Adding instability.** Place an unstable surface (pillow, rolled-up towel, or balance disc) underneath the foot of your back leg.

4. Alternating Quad Stretch

Make it more manageable by:

- **Holding on to something.** Just like with the Standing Hamstring and Nerve Floss Stretch, I prefer that you don't use any form of support. If you absolutely can't do the exercise without help, then use a wall or the edge of a table, but work toward weaning yourself off these supports.

Elevate the intensity by:

- **Adding instability.** Stand with both feet on an unstable surface (pillow, rolled-up towel, or two balance discs).
- **Closing one eye.** Your body has to work even harder to stabilize itself when you apply this trick, which you can do several ways.

You could try closing one eye for half of the repetitions, then closing the other eye for the remaining reps. Or close whichever eye is on the same side of the foot you're raising behind you (or close the opposite eye—left eye/right foot or right eye/left foot).

5. Single-Arm Pectoral Stretch

Make it more manageable by:

- **Lowering your arm slightly.** If you feel any pain in your elbow when performing this movement, moving your elbow an inch or two lower can minimize discomfort.

Elevate the intensity by:

- **Holding the stretch a little longer.** Instead of 3 to 5 seconds, shoot for 6 to 10 seconds to give your chest, shoulders, and neck more attention.

6. Angel Stretch

Make it more manageable by:

- **Working with your body.** If you're curvaceous, your backside might cause you to have problems getting everything to touch the wall (head, upper back, elbows, backs of your hands, and heels). If that's the case, try tilting your pelvis forward and hold it in that position.
- **Grabbing a few towels.** If that still doesn't fix the problem (or you lack the mobility in your hips for now), place a few rolled-up towels behind your head and upper back so that you have some contact with the wall. Your heels and elbows might not touch, but don't force them back to make them. So long as your fingernails are touching the wall, that's fine for now.

- **Not getting discouraged.** The good news is, the more you do the program, the more your hip and lower spine mobility will improve. That additional flexibility will make it easier for you to tilt your pelvis forward and backward, allowing you to adjust yourself more effectively so that you can touch everything without any issues.

Elevate the intensity by:

- **Opening up the stretch.** Put a large foam roller behind you (perpendicular to the floor) so that everything from your head down to your tailbone is resting on it. Again, you won't have full contact with the wall (your elbows and heels specifically), but this variation further opens up your chest and shoulders.

7. On-the-Floor Marching

Make it more manageable by:

- **Shortening the movement.** Instead of sweeping your arms all the way behind you and bringing your knees up until your thigh is perpendicular to the floor, try moving them half the distance.
- **Not being hard on yourself.** Look, this one takes a little coordination, which means even if you have a decent fitness base, you might still struggle with this movement because it requires some synchronicity. Be patient and it will come with time.

Elevate the intensity by:

- **Adding instability.** Something I do every day with LeBron is have him do this move lying back lengthwise on a long foam roller (positioned from his head, down his spine, and stopping at his tailbone). You'll need to bend your legs slightly (instead of keeping them perfectly straight), but beyond that, you'll perform the move as described.

8. On-the-Floor Pilates 100

Make it more manageable by:

- **Slowing things down.** Try adjusting the tempo until you find a pace that feels just right for your current fitness level.

Elevate the intensity by:

- **Raising your legs.** Keeping your knees bent, lift your legs up so that your thighs are perpendicular to the floor and hold them there for the duration of the movement.
- **Adding leg kicks.** After every 5 pulses, pause, then quickly extend your left leg out and back, then quickly extend your right leg out and back—without moving your head, upper body, or arms.

9. Glute Bridge

Make it more manageable by:

- **Not going up as high.** If raising your hips up until your body forms a straight line is too taxing (for now), try lifting yourself up about halfway—or even just an inch or two from the floor. Even the slightest motion will strengthen your muscles, allowing you to become more efficient with the movement over time.

Elevate the intensity by:

- **Pulsing at the top.** After you pause at the top for 3 seconds, add a few extra pulses in between every repetition by dropping your hips an inch or so, then raising them a few times (2 to 3 is fine) before lowering yourself back down to the floor.
- **Trying it one leg at a time.** Instead of keeping both feet on the floor, try a "single-leg glute bridge" by starting with both feet flat

on the floor, then extending one leg straight out—keeping your thighs parallel to each other—before starting the exercise. Do the same number of repetitions for each leg.

10. Push-Up

Make it more manageable by:

- **Resting on your knees.** If you can't do a traditional push-up, you can drop to your knees.
- **Not going down as far.** Instead of bending your elbows and lowering yourself until your upper arms are parallel to the floor, try to go down a third to half the distance and then slowly push yourself back up.
- **Being negative–in a good way.** Instead of slowly pushing yourself up and lowering yourself down, focus on the lowering portion only. Once you've reached the ground, instead of pushing yourself back up, just get back up into position doing whatever you need to do. Trust me—you're still working your body using what is known as eccentric (or negative) training, which will allow you to build up strength and endurance so that eventually you can perform the exercise as described.

Elevate the intensity by:

- **Pausing at the midpoint.** Each time you're halfway down or halfway back up, pause for a second or two. All your muscles—especially your core—will be screaming at you.
- **Slowing things down further.** If you can do more than 15 repetitions, don't add more. Instead, try slowing the movement down. Find a pace that allows you to do only between 8 to 15 repetitions before your muscles feel too fatigued to continue.

- **Adding some instability.** Place the tops of your feet up on a balance disc—or put each hand on a balance disc instead of the floor. Either variation will make it more difficult for you to maintain your balance.
- **Moving your hands closer.** Bringing your fingertips and thumbs together (so they form a diamond shape) not only shifts more emphasis to your triceps, but it requires more effort from your core and proprioceptive muscles to stay balanced.
- **Getting a leg up.** Each time LeBron lowers himself to the floor, he raises one foot off the ground up toward the ceiling, keeping his leg straight as he goes. As he presses himself back up, he lowers his foot back to the floor (alternating back and forth from his left leg to his right leg with each push-up). This variation brings in more posterior core and glute activation.

11. Bent-Knee Side Plank

Make it more manageable by:

- **Holding the movement for less time.** Instead of pausing for 5 seconds at the top, experiment with less—going down to even 1 second if necessary—and build up to 5.
- **Skipping the pause entirely.** If you struggle with being able to hold yourself at the top for even 1 second, then just do the movement up and down at a controlled pace (not fast!). You'll quickly build up strength and endurance as you stick with the program, which will allow you to eventually hold yourself at the top much easier.

Elevate the intensity by:

- **Adding some instability.** You can change the surface by placing a rolled-up towel or exercise disc under your elbow or knee (or both!) on the ground.

- **Loading on a little weight.** If you have at least 6 months of exercise under your belt—and have someone who can safely assist you—then you could have them put (and hold) an exercise plate directly on top of your hip.

[**NOTE:** Some trainers might have you straighten the bottom leg closest to the floor, which is something I don't advocate. Does that make the move harder? Yes, but for the wrong reason in that it compromises your lower back by putting unnecessary stress on it. LeBron has one of the strongest cores of any athlete I've ever seen—and he only does this exercise with his bottom leg bent.]

12. Side Plank with Leg Raise

Make it more manageable by:

- **Dropping the plank.** If you're having a hard time either strength- or endurance-wise, skip the plank altogether and lie down on your side—then perform just the leg raise.
- **Tapping your foot.** The reason I asked you not to let your foot of the leg you're raising up and down touch the floor is that it creates a "micro-rest" for your muscles instead of keeping them engaged the entire time. If you need that rest to complete the movement, then use it (but try to reduce how often you touch the floor as you progress).

Elevate the intensity by:

- **Slowing things down further.** Instead of moving at a 3-seconds-up/ 3-seconds-down tempo, experiment with raising and lowering your leg at a much slower speed.
- **Adding some instability.** You can change the surface by placing a rolled-up towel or exercise disc under your elbow or knee (or both!) on the ground.
- **Strapping on some weight.** Some overachieving clients (my warriors!) wonder if adding leg weights to their ankles would be

helpful. Can you do it? Yes. But I feel the suggestions above are equally effective and a lot safer. Attaching an ankle weight will only serve to overload your body with weight far from your core, and in my opinion it isn't as practical, particularly because it increases your risk of injury. But if you feel that you're ready and choose to do it, stick with a weight under 5 pounds.

13. Side Plank March

Make it more manageable by:

- **Shortening the range of motion.** Don't swing your leg and arm as far back behind you and in front of you as you can. This will minimize some of the motion that could be making it more difficult for you to stay balanced or coordinated.

Elevate the intensity by:

- **Adding some instability.** Again, you can change the surface by placing a rolled-up towel or exercise disc under your elbow or knee (or both!) on the ground.
- **Strapping on some weight.** If you've been working out at least 6 months, you can add an ankle weight to your leg, but don't exceed 2½ pounds.

14. Traditional Plank

Make it more manageable by:

- **Planking for less time.** Instead of striving for 15 to 20 seconds, just hold the pose for as long as you're able.
- **Changing your base slightly.** Instead of having your feet together, space them farther apart from each other, which will make it easier for you to stabilize yourself.

Elevate the intensity by:

- **Seeing how long you can hold it.** You could shoot beyond the 15 to 20 seconds I'm recommending, but don't go beyond 2 minutes. You won't reap any additional benefit by doing so. Plus, it might lengthen the workout in a way that makes you rush through the back half.
- **Strapping on some weight.** You can have someone gently put a weight plate on your lower back or butt, so long as it never compromises your stability or technique.

15. Superman

Make it more manageable by:

- **Pausing for less time.** Instead of holding yourself up for 3 to 5 seconds, do it for only 1 or 2 seconds, or skip the pause altogether and just slowly raise yourself up and down.
- **Leaving your legs down.** Instead of raising your arms and legs together, lift only your upper body off the floor.
- **Bending your arms at 90 degrees.** The farther your arms are extended away from your body, the more challenging the movement is on your muscles. By bending your arms, you're creating an angle that reduces the resistance slightly.

Elevate the intensity by:

- **Pausing longer at the top.** If you're looking for more of a challenge, try holding the position for a few more seconds.
- **Raising one arm and one leg at a time.** This variation takes a little coordination, but try raising (then lowering) your left arm and right leg together, then switching arms and legs. The movement should feel like you're swimming. This tweak causes your body to rock back and forth more, which forces your proprioceptive muscles to work even harder to stabilize you.

16. Alternating Arm/Leg Raise

Make it more manageable by:

- **Supporting your torso.** If you can find a footrest, chair, bench, or some other sturdy object that allows you to position yourself over the top of it so that you can rest your chest on it—but still allows your hands and knees to touch the floor—give it a try.
- **Skipping the pause.** Instead of holding the move at the top, just go up and down at a controlled pace.

Elevate the intensity by:

- **Lying over a stability ball.** Technically, you're doing the same thing—supporting your torso—by draping yourself over a stability ball. But its shape makes it harder for you to maintain balance.
- **Closing your eyes—or just one.** Either way, it adds another level of difficulty to the movement.
- **Balancing yourself on your fingers and toes.** Instead of keeping your palms and knees on the floor, raise your knees just off the floor so that you're supported by only your toes—then adjust your hands so that you're up on your fingertips.

17. Kneeling Hip Hinge

Make it more manageable by:

- **Not lowering down as much.** Instead of tilting your hips all the way back so that your butt reaches your heels, only tilt your hips half as far.
- **Not bending over as much.** Instead of bending at the waist until your torso is at a 45-degree angle, try cutting the distance you lean forward in half.

Elevate the intensity by:

- **Widening your range.** If you can do it without toppling over or compromising your lower back, lower yourself farther than 45 degrees.
- **Straightening your arms.** Raise your arms straight up over your head, then keep them in line with your torso the entire time.
- **Raising yourself higher.** Position yourself on a weight bench—or place two sturdy chairs of equal size next to each other and kneel on them instead (one knee on each chair)—to add an unstable component to the movement.

18. Single-Leg Hip Hinge

Make it more manageable by:

- **Lowering down less.** Instead of tilting your hips all the way back so that your butt reaches your heels, tilt your hips only half as far.
- **Bending over less.** Instead of bending at the waist until your torso is at a 45-degree angle, try cutting the distance you lean forward in half.

Elevate the intensity by:

- **Adding instability.** Tuck a balance disc or foam roller underneath your knee.
- **Dropping yourself down even farther.** If you can do it without losing your balance or straining your lower back, lower yourself farther than 45 degrees.
- **Straightening your arms.** Raise your arms straight up over your head, then keep them in line with your torso the entire time.

19. Ankle-Tap Downward Dog

Make it more manageable by:

- **Not reaching back as far.** Even though touching your ankles is the goal, tapping your kneecaps—or just reaching back as far as you comfortably can—will still work until your mobility and balance improves with time.

Elevate the intensity by:

- **Bringing your feet closer together.** The more you shorten the distance between your feet, the harder it is to maintain your balance.

20. Spider-Man Stretch

Make it more manageable by:

- **Being comfortable with your range.** If you can't get your foot up to your hand, stick with half the distance for now.
- **Elevating yourself.** Instead of having your hands on the floor in a push-up position, place them on the seat of a sturdy chair. This tweak removes much of the upper-body effort and makes it more of a lower-body exercise.

Elevate the intensity by:

- **Bending your arms slightly.** Keeping your elbows partially bent throughout the movement forces your chest, shoulders, triceps, and core muscles to stay contracted to keep you upright.
- **Doing push-ups in between.** After you've planted your feet twice (left foot, then right foot), try performing 1 or 2 push-ups, then repeat.

21. Standing Pelvic Tilt & 22. Thoracic Spine Rotation

These two movements belong together because they're probably the easiest ones to do, so they don't require easier modifications. Your hips and thoracic spine are going to move only as far as you presently have mobility in them—and pushing them beyond what you can comfortably do would only bring more harm than good. That said, both are minimal movements that can make a major impact on your overall performance—if you take both seriously.

They're also not moves that I ever encourage intensifying in any way, even if that were possible. Could you do more repetitions? Theoretically, yes, but these are two pieces of a much larger puzzle, a series of movements meant to prepare your body from head to toe. Going overboard with tilting your pelvis and rotating your shoulders a hundred times each isn't going to take anything to another level, so I want you to save that time and enthusiasm for the rest of the program.

23. Single-Leg Balance Oscillation

Make it more manageable by:

- **Holding on to something.** You can grab a wall, the edge of a table, a sturdy chair, or any object that won't budge on you.

Elevate the intensity by:

- **Adding some instability.** You can change the surface by standing on a rolled-up towel or exercise disc.
- **Strapping on some weight.** If you have at least 6 months of working out under your belt, you can add an ankle weight to your extended leg, but don't exceed 2½ pounds.

24. Sumo Lateral Squat

Make it more manageable by:

- **Standing a few inches away from a wall.** By positioning yourself with your back as close to a sturdy wall as possible, if you lose your balance, you'll gently lean against the wall and catch yourself.
- **Using your arms to counterbalance.** Instead of keeping your hands in front of your chest, start with your arms hanging down in front of you (not by your sides so that they don't interfere with the exercise). As you squat down, swing them forward to help stabilize you, then lower them as you press yourself back up.

Elevate the intensity by:

- **Closing one eye—or both.** You could try closing one eye for half of the repetitions, then close the other eye for the remaining reps. Or close whichever eye is on the same side of the leg you're bending (or close the opposite eye—left eye/right leg or right eye/left leg).
- **Adding some weight.** Try holding a dumbbell or weight plate with both hands in front of your chest or grab a dumbbell in each hand and let your arms hang straight down at your sides.

25. Split-Stance Isometric Wall Squat

Make it more manageable by:

- **Holding the position for less time.** Instead of 20 seconds, just maintain the pose for as long as you can.
- **Not going down as deep.** Ideally, you should strive to squat down until your thigh is parallel to the floor. But if you can only lower yourself a few inches for now, take the win and challenge yourself to go an inch farther the next time.

Elevate the intensity by:

- **Holding the position for more time.** You can go beyond 20 seconds and hold the move for up to 1 minute, but don't go beyond that.
- **Adding some instability.** You can change the surface by standing on a rolled-up towel or exercise disc. Or put a stability ball behind you and hold it in place against the wall with whichever foot would typically be flat against the wall.

26. Single-Leg Romanian Deadlift (RDL)

Make it more manageable by:

- **Not going down as far.** This move takes balance, so if you can't perform it as described, just lower your torso down as far as you comfortably can.

Elevate the intensity by:

- **Closing your eyes.** This makes the move even more difficult by challenging your proprioception.
- **Adding some weight.** Only after you've mastered the move would I recommend either holding one dumbbell (with either hand) or holding a pair of dumbbells (with one in each hand). As you do the move, just let your arms hang straight down.

27. Rocket Ship

Make it more manageable by:

- **Holding the position for less time.** If 2 or 3 seconds is too difficult, just hold the pose as long as possible.
- **Grabbing on to something.** If you're having a difficult time getting up into position, you can use one hand to hold on to a nearby chair, table, or anything sturdy to support yourself.

Elevate the intensity by:

- **Adding some instability.** You can change the surface by standing on a rolled-up towel, two balance discs, or a few pillows.
- **Closing your eyes.** As much as I prefer you looking up at the sky or ceiling because this final move is so empowering, I can't argue that doing it with your eyes closed definitely tests your balance—so try it out!

Sit Less–Stride More

Hold on . . . you're not done yet. If you're coming to this regimen as a person who isn't super active, you may need to make a lot of these modifications at first to make certain exercises and stretches more manageable. Don't worry, though—it won't take long before your body adjusts and becomes more competent with the routine, but there's also one other thing you can be doing to speed that transition, and it's super simple—it's get moving!

Like I said, my mobility routine can be added on top of anything:

- It works alongside any workout program that you want to get more from, whether that's circuit training, strength training, powerlifting, bodybuilding—it doesn't really matter what your individual goals might be.
- It works together with any sport or activity you're presently doing.
- It works as a standalone, helping you perform even the most mundane of tasks more efficiently throughout the day. But, if that's you, then I need you to do something for me. Actually, let me rephrase that: I need you to do something for yourself.

My program is designed for you to get more from your body for as long as possible. But if you're presently not doing anything for your body—particularly from a cardiovascular standpoint—then I can't promise you peak performance at the same level that you're hoping for. If right now you're not exercising or participating in a sport on a regular basis—at least three times weekly for at least twenty minutes—then I need you to move.

Sit less and stride more. Literally two things anyone can do that collectively impact your health in ways that you may not give them credit for. Sure, I work with high-caliber athletes, but I also work with celebrities and other people who honestly don't have the time to do much more than my mobility program. And when I look at how their day breaks out, I really can't disagree with them. But in those instances—just like right now with you—I immediately point out how no matter what type of busy day they're having:

- **They have the power to stand instead of sit.**
- **They have the power to move instead of stand.**

Stand Up for Yourself

It's honestly not rocket science to say that the less time you spend in a seated position, the more often your body is burning a few more calories (.15 more per minute standing than sitting[1]) and lowering your risk of health issues, including heart disease, cancer, and diabetes. Equally important, sitting more can cause postural problems that can impact your mobility and performance, as well as increase your risk of injuring yourself. And yet, the average American adult sits six and a half hours a day[2]—and out of that group, one in four adults park their butt more than eight hours daily.

Simply put, sitting is bad for you. Need a few examples? How about the fact that sitting more than two hours a day watching TV raises your chances of experiencing young-onset colorectal cancer by 70 percent,[3] or the fact that sitting has been shown to thin out portions of your brain linked to memory?[4] Research has even shown that sitting more than ten hours a day can affect you on a cellular level, making certain cells biologically as much as eight years older than your actual age.[5]

Reversing those risks is literally as easy as making yourself vertical as often as possible all day long. Sure, sometimes sitting is unavoidable, especially during mealtime, when traveling, or other moments when it's either awkward or impossible to not plant yourself in a seat. But generally, you do have a choice. By choosing to stand instead of sit, you're not coasting through life—you're conquering it.

How to Pull It Off Painlessly

First, own your inactivity. At least once a week, pull out your phone and open the stopwatch feature. Hit Start every time you sit down and Stop every time you get up. We need that baseline for how often you're seated daily. Each week, repeat this exercise but try to shave off a few minutes from your previous time.

Put a reminder within view. It's not really your fault for sitting as much as you do. Many of the activities we do seated—channel surfing, working a desk job, watching a game—are designed to draw our attention away. Putting something that reminds you to stand nearby—something visible that you can't escape seeing at least every minute—can be a game-changer. In fact, research has shown that using some form of prompt to remind you to stand is extremely effective at changing sedentary behavior.[6]

Anything will work—Post-it notes (or even a piece of painter's tape) on your computer, couch, kitchen chair—wherever you spend any time sitting. Make the background of your phone a picture of your kids standing up, or put your phone on vibrate and set the timer to go off every few minutes. If you're self-conscious about making it that obvious, just put a Band-Aid on your finger so that every time you see or feel it, you'll be reminded that it stands for, well, standing up!

This reminder need not even be tangible; it can be connected to an activity. Are you texting or emailing every five minutes? Then make a rule never to sit when responding to someone. Watch a lot of TV or YouTube? Stand during every commercial break or sit when you're searching but stand once you hit Play. Always checking social media, the time, or weather updates on your phone? Don't do it unless you're standing upright—then make a point to stay that way for at least 3 to 5 minutes afterward.

We all have bad habits, things we find ourselves doing way more often than we should. Using these tricks can turn them into healthy opportunities.

Walk It Off

If you don't presently exercise, I need you to at least do a minimum of 150 minutes of cardiovascular exercise each week. That's the magic number that decades-worth of science has shown can help you extend your longevity by decreasing your risk of many chronic diseases and medical conditions, such as cancer, diabetes, and hypertension. That precise amount of activity plays a part in strengthening your heart, managing your weight, keeping your blood pressure nice and stable, and preventing you from being at risk of metabolic syndrome,[7] a group of risk factors that can make you more susceptible to cardiovascular disease, among other things. In fact, it's been shown that at least 150 minutes of moderate-intensity activity each week could increase your lifespan by as much as five years.[8]

Now, could you get those 150 minutes riding a bike, swimming in a pool, or jumping on a rowing machine? Sure, you could, but if you're not doing anything at all right now, chances are these ways of breaking a sweat are either not interesting or not available to you.

That's where walking comes in. This simple activity, which we start doing as toddlers and don't often even think of as an *activity*, has a lot going for it:

- It's excuse-proof. It doesn't require special equipment and can be done anywhere.
- It works the same muscles as running (your quadriceps, hamstrings, glutes, calves, abdominals, and lower back), but with less stress on your joints.
- It has been shown to be effective at improving your body's ability to consume oxygen, raising high-density lipoprotein (HDL) cholesterol, and lowering blood pressure[9] and low-density lipoprotein (LDL) cholesterol. In fact, research shows that when we're moving about, we tend to feel better mentally and less stressed.[10]

- It's one of the few versions of cardio you can do in reverse. By walking backward (either outside, on a treadmill, or even up a staircase) at a slower pace than you otherwise would (for safety reasons), you're not just making things more interesting for yourself. This subtle tweak utilizes more of your quadriceps and reduces sheer force on your kneecaps (which helps strengthen your knees to make them more injury-resistant), in addition to stimulating your central nervous system and improving your balance and coordination.
- Finally, it's one of the most versatile forms of cardiovascular exercise. You can effortlessly raise or lower the intensity by changing your tempo or by adding extra resistance, such as wearing boots or a rucksack, walking in tall grass or waist-high water, or just holding a light dumbbell in each hand. You can change the angle of the surface you're walking on (straight, incline, or decline) or even change the surface altogether (macadam, trails, hills, sand, and so on).

How to Pull It Off Painlessly

For this one, you have a choice: You can concentrate on doing 150 minutes of walking at a moderate-intensity per week (broken up into five thirty-minute sessions). Or you can just go about your day (and not bother with finding time for five walking workouts). However, you must walk at least 10,000 steps a day.

If you choose the first option: I need you walking at a pace that keeps your heart rate elevated between 50 to 70 percent of your maximum heart rate (or MHR) and keeping it at that level for the entire duration. What's your MHR? Just subtract your age from 220. For example, if you're 40, then your MHR would be 180 (220 – 40 = 180).

Using a heart-rate monitor will help you stay in that zone, but another way you can tell if you're exercising at a moderate intensity is to open your mouth and try to have a conversation:

- If you can speak long sentences without feeling out of breath, you're probably at a pace that has your pulse below 50 percent of your MHR—so crank it up.
- If you can talk but singing would be impossible, your pulse is most likely between 50 to 70 percent of your MHR. Walking at a pace of between 110 to 120 steps per minute is fast enough to do the trick for most people.
- If you're unable to talk and walk, you're pushing yourself too hard and probably have a pulse above 70 percent of your MHR—so dial it back.

If you choose the second option: Then you're going to need a few things.

1. A **water-resistant pedometer** (or fitness tracker) to track your steps. Can you use the activity tracker on your phone? You can, but even if you're the type that has their phone on them all the time, there might be moments during the day when it's not, and I prefer that you're accountable for every step. If high-tech monitoring is what you're looking for, I highly recommend using a WHOOP Health Monitor.
2. If you don't have a **Bluetooth headset**, invest in one. What I don't want you to have is anything that prevents you from moving from one spot to another. Unless you live in Minnesota and it's wintertime, there's literally no excuse not to be able to walk around the parking lot or outside your house whenever you're taking a phone call.

WITH ALL THE STEPS NOW in place to keep you moving, it's time to begin laying the foundation on how to help your body heal itself even faster and more efficiently than ever before.

PART III

MEND

CHAPTER 11

Think It Forward

When I start working with a new client and running them through the paces, I look at a lot of things. Sometimes, even though they are putting in the work when it comes to exercise and diet, I can tell that something is *off.*

My program is designed to facilitate recovery, so when a client doesn't seem to be bouncing back quickly or efficiently, I start probing to see if what's happening behind the curtain is adversely affecting their performance on the stage of life. Together, we re-examine both the obvious and hidden aspects of their day (and night) to look for potential problems. I learned this lesson early in my career and made it my mantra: ***Recovery never stops—unless you decide it does.***

But what exactly *is* recovery? The term has become a catchphrase that everyone uses but nobody quite gets. Most label it under *rest*—rest after exercise, rest after a long day at work or raising the kids, or rest after an injury or illness. Others tie it to practices that can aid in healing, such as massage, cryo baths, and other therapeutic techniques. But very few fully understand how far-reaching recovery really is.

Recovery isn't just about grabbing a heating pad. Instead, it's asking yourself: *"How quickly can I bounce back to achieve the same level of performance that I accomplished yesterday—and maybe even a little better?"*

It really doesn't matter what you do for a living or what your goals are. Whether you're an elite athlete or an armchair quarterback, a stressed-out stockbroker or a stay-at-home dad, it's about taking the necessary steps that allow you to regenerate while still maintaining a high level of performance from your body. It's about rewinding yourself today by focusing on resting your mind and body, as well as relieving both of stress, so that you can hit the fast-forward button tomorrow. Recovery is crucial but often doesn't get the attention it deserves, for a few reasons:

We believe we're falling behind if we stop moving. We live in a society that admires and rewards hard work, which makes it difficult to embrace the notion that taking the time to relax—even if it's just for a few minutes—could actually be a good thing. It's important to be driven, and I work with some of the most determined people on the planet. But what got them to where they are isn't just their strength of will, but their understanding that to succeed continuously, you must remind yourself that it happens only if you also take time to stop and destress once in a while.

It can sometimes feel counterproductive to allow yourself downtime, especially when you're in the middle of something incredibly important. It can seem like a huge mistake putting certain things on pause to give yourself time to heal. The good news is, if that's you, I've found that people who fit this category—those compelled to sacrifice in order to succeed—usually stop feeling that way once they learn through experience how valuable downtime can be. They understand how rest and recovery allow them to accomplish even more because if you're looking to cross that finish line a winner, then giving your body time to heal is the only way to make that victory possible.

We feel selfish for allowing ourselves to breathe. I don't know what's happening in your world right now, but I'm certain there's a lot going on. Have you ever met somebody who wasn't busy? I haven't, but I don't think it's because my job is training high-performing individuals—it's just how life works. It can be hard to think about ourselves when we're busy taking care of others. Maybe you're a parent trying to juggle a full-time job and a family, or a person who is responsible for so much that the thought of stepping away from those obligations for even a moment is laughable—not necessarily because you don't have the time in the day to do it, but because it wouldn't feel right to do it.

I'm guilty of thinking this way myself. As a father and a husband, one who spends a lot of time on the road for my job, any free time I have when not working gets directed toward my family because they are always my top priority. I need to remind myself perpetually about the importance of recovery, particularly rejuvenation techniques that require a little "me time." I know that certain steps that may seem to cut into my family time actually improve that time by enabling me to be energetic and present when I'm with them.

We take a certain pride in suffering. There's a sense of unnecessary shame that sometimes gets in the way of rest and recovery. A lot of us have been taught to not admit certain things because if we do, we're somehow weaker. We're taught to act like soldiers and not sufferers.

For example, when was the last time you were exhausted—both physically and mentally—but didn't want to admit it because you thought it would make you seem old? Or the last time you pushed yourself a little too hard when exercising or playing a sport, but came to work the next day pretending your back wasn't killing you—all because you didn't want to seem like a lightweight?

At some point, we've all pushed past pain and fatigue, not just because we wanted to avoid seeming weak, but because it made us feel even stronger. This is where it gets tricky. You see, I would never tell you *not* to overcome obstacles, because that's how you can move forward. However, it's important to heed what your body is trying to tell you.

What to Think Through . . .

Before Starting This Program

Will You Be Comfortable—Making Yourself Comfortable?

Here's the deal: I need you in the right headspace before you implement any of these recovery recommendations. So if the words *bath*, *massage*, or *nap* sound passive, lazy, or ridiculous, you need to shake those thoughts out of your mind right now or you'll never achieve what you're fully capable of.

To motivate you to stay the course, I could go on and tell you how you're worth it, how you deserve to treat yourself, and other things like that, which would all be true. But instead, I would rather remind you how not only are these mending methods incredibly important components of my program, but they're also used by my clients and many high performers on a regular basis.

You need to go into this program understanding that what might feel self-indulgent or silly is what sustains peak performance. In other words, remind yourself that the fact that they feel good in the first place proves they're doing their job in helping your body heal and recover.

Will You Be Comfortable—Making Yourself Uncomfortable?

Look, not everything I'll be sharing with you in the next few chapters is going to be a walk in the park. There will be suggestions that will take some getting used to, and some that might feel like major sacrifices: going to bed earlier than usual, monitoring your nicotine or alcohol consumption, or stepping away from certain things prior to bedtime. There will be others (ice baths, anyone?) that are downright brutal. But know this: Nothing I'll be suggesting would be a part of my program if it didn't pay off in the end.

You need to ask yourself how much your own longevity is worth to you. Is being able to perform at your absolute best for as long as possible worth a little inconvenience or discomfort?

Those at the top of their game already know the answer to that question because they understand that staying on top is about having the willpower and guts to do what it takes to keep their body in a constant state of healing. They may not understand all the nuts and bolts that are necessary to achieve this, but in a moment you will have that knowledge. So do you have what it takes to keep your body in a constant state of healing?

What to Think Through . . .

Before Every Mending Session

As I mentioned earlier, in order to create an environment that allows you to heal faster and more efficiently, you need to be smarter when it comes to how you *rest* and *relieve* both your body and your mind. But before you use any of the tactics I'm going to suggest, you'll need to do another self-diagnosis similar to the quick questionnaires I recommended in both the Eat and Move sections.

How Do You Feel in *This* Moment?

One hour before bedtime. You should have a baseline on a few key questions:

1. **How hard did you push yourself physically today?**
   (1 being not at all; 10 being to the brink of exhaustion):
   1 2 3 4 5 6 7 8 9 10
2. **How hard did you push yourself mentally today?**
   (1 being not at all; 10 being to the absolute extreme):
   1 2 3 4 5 6 7 8 9 10
3. **Where would you rank your stress level?**
   (1 being completely chill; 10 being seriously distressed):
   1 2 3 4 5 6 7 8 9 10
4. **Finally, how tired do you feel right now?**
   (1 being not at all; 10 being barely staying awake):
   1 2 3 4 5 6 7 8 9 10

Now, why am I asking you to answer these *one hour* before bedtime instead of waiting until your head hits the pillow? Sometimes considering these questions can make your mind a bit more active. Thinking about these questions an hour out (give or take—you don't have to be precise) won't affect your answers one bit but can keep you from accidentally self-sabotaging your sleep.

Before any other tactic in the next chapter. Even though the suggestions I'll be making may be different from one another, you'll still be able to assess their overall effectiveness by considering the following questions prior to taking any of them on:

1. **Where would you rank your energy level?**
   (1 being the least alert; 10 being the most alert):
   1 2 3 4 5 6 7 8 9 10
2. **How calm do you feel right now?**
   (1 being not at all; 10 being as relaxed as possible):
   1 2 3 4 5 6 7 8 9 10
3. **How would you rank how achy/sore/tight you feel overall (head to toe)?**
   (1 being not at all; 10 being in serious pain):
   1 2 3 4 5 6 7 8 9 10

NOW THAT YOU'VE TAKEN A few things into account, it's time to take control of how fast and how fully you recover—so get ready to recharge!

CHAPTER 12

Follow It Through

Recovery goes hand in hand with nutrition and exercise, and together they are the three crucial players that help you stay in the game longer. In other words, how you're eating and how you're moving also affect how well you're mending. Certain nutrients are providing your body what it needs to repair itself while certain movements are improving blood-flow circulation to make sure those nutrients get where they're needed most—helping you heal. But the healing doesn't stop there.

I'm a huge believer that recovery shouldn't start after performance but during performance. During games, I'm on the sidelines sitting right behind LeBron's chair so whenever he comes off the court, I'm there at the ready, communicating both verbally and nonverbally as to how he's doing and feeling—no different from how an F1 race engineer is in constant communication with their driver during a race. So, for example, in my mind, I'm starting LeBron's recovery in the third quarter, maximizing time-outs and doing little things on the bench that I know will ease his joints and prep his body for a late-game push. Then, when the fourth quarter comes around—boom! He's able to let loose and kill it. And once the game is over, we're busy that night implementing everything necessary to recover so he's able to reach that same level of performance the next day.

Now it's your turn to consider a few recovery-accelerating choices that will extend your longevity by helping promote the healing process, both day and night.

The Rules of the Regimen

This is going to sound simple at first, and that's exactly my hope: that you will recognize just how easy it is to stay in a constant state of healing and how it doesn't take much to get the ball rolling and keep it in motion. In fact, it might be *because* this seems so easy to do that a lot of people don't bother doing it—because what's easy and feels good can't possibly be effective, right? That's not going to be you. Instead, you're going to try to adhere to the following blueprint every single day:

- **Get between seven and eight hours of high-quality sleep.**
- **Soothe your muscles and/or mind with at least one form of recuperative therapy.**
- **Take a few deep breaths at least once every hour.**

Doesn't sound so difficult, does it? But if you really think about it, when was the last time you did all three in the same day? I'll say that again: When was the last time you got enough sleep, took the time to focus on your breathing, and enjoyed some form of therapeutic treatment that brought relief to your entire body—all in the same day?

Exactly.

I'm willing to bet there are a lot of readers of this book—and maybe you're one of them—that have never done all three in one day. And even if you're one of those rare few that has pulled off this hat trick in the past, I'm willing to bet you didn't repeat the trifecta the next day, despite how much better it made you feel. Perhaps you didn't fully appreciate how each of these mending motivators were working behind the scenes to make you feel like a million bucks.

So let's get into the how and why these three things are so important.

Get Between Seven and Eight Hours of High-Quality Sleep

There's a reason you feel great after a good night's sleep. While you were at rest, other parts of you were hard at work to make sure you came back as strong as possible today.

During sleep your immune system finally gets the time to focus on its many tasks, which includes eliminating viruses and other pathogens. It's also triggering the release of certain things such as T-cells (white blood cells),[1] in addition to growth hormones to stave off infection. The same goes for your muscles, all of which use that uninterrupted time to heal themselves, fiber by fiber. On top of it all, getting a solid night's sleep has been shown to significantly reduce chronic inflammation. When you choose to not snooze, not only do you lose out on these and other benefits, but you also put your longevity at risk in many frightening ways.

For example, losing just a few hours of sleep has been shown to induce inflammation.[2] In fact, research has shown that lack of sleep elevates both interleukin-6 and C-reactive protein in the blood,[3] both of which are tied to severe age-related issues, including hypertension, cardiovascular issues, and type-2 diabetes. Everything from elevating your blood pressure[4] to inhibiting your brain's ability to learn and memorize[5]—even making you crave more calories[6] and sugar[7]—has been proven to be tied to not getting enough shut-eye. This is why I take sleep so seriously. And not just any sleep—but the best rest possible.

Every night, you switch between two forms of sleep: the first is non-rapid eye movement sleep (NREM), which begins when you fall asleep and lasts for about ninety minutes. The second is rapid eye movement sleep (REM), and it's during this state when you do most of your dreaming, your eyes begin to move quickly, and you start twitching. REM doesn't last long, about ten minutes the first time through it. After that, your body begins a new sleep cycle, shifting back to NREM for another ninety minutes before returning to REM sleep once again, this time for a few minutes longer.

But here's the thing: The body heals and repairs itself at an optimal level when it's in REM sleep—or "dream sleep"—and the longer you can remain in REM sleep, the more recharged and refreshed you'll feel the next day. On the flip side, of course, the less sleep you allow yourself, the fewer sleep cycles you'll experience. And even if you're the type that always gets eight hours, you could still be missing out. REM sleep occurs only at the end of every sleep cycle, so the more often you're disturbed during the night, the more likely you're missing out on entering REM sleep as often as you should be, since every disruption starts the cycle all over again (beginning with NREM sleep).

Simply put, there is no way to get back to 100 percent as quickly as possible—both physically and emotionally—if you cannot experience as much REM sleep as possible. So you need to take sleep seriously. Now I'm going to get you to that place much faster—and stay in that zone longer—so you enjoy more time to heal throughout the night.

The Optimal Sleep Anytime Blueprint

When I'm on the road with LeBron, we're moving from town to town, every hotel room pretty much different from the last. It's the type of schedule most would find maddening if trying to get a good night's sleep is your goal. It's not always easy to relax when you're resting your head in a place that's unfamiliar, something I'm sure you've experienced before while on vacation or traveling for work. But when my client's performance depends on their ability to heal during the night, I can't afford to have them experience a poor night's sleep.

You're about to discover my *Optimal Sleep Anytime Blueprint*, which allows LeBron and others to always fall into a deep REM sleep faster and for longer. By implementing this precise sleep-enhancing routine every night, their bodies get exactly what they need to heal and recharge, no matter where they find themselves when on the road. But better still, this routine's even more effective when you're staying put in your own bed and have even less distractions to contend with. It works like this:

One hour before bedtime

Dim all lights to as low as possible. Darkness is king when it comes to inducing sleep, which means the sooner you can bring the lights down, the better. Exposure to artificial light between dusk and bedtime significantly suppresses melatonin—a hormone produced at night by the pineal gland in your brain that's not only responsible for regulating your sleep-wake cycle, but also helps lower your blood pressure and body temperature.

Lower the temperature to 68°F or below. With LeBron, we bring the room temperature down to this level, and I like to start the process an hour before bedtime just in case it takes longer than usual to cool things down. Why this cool? Research shows that lowering your body's internal core temperature helps to maintain circadian rhythms and improve sleep quality.

Now, some experts will argue that you should go even lower. Some believe 65°F is the magic number, while others suggest going as low as 60°F. You can experiment as you like, so long as the temperature never rises above 68°F.

Thirty minutes before bedtime

Cut off all screen time. That includes tablets, TVs, and, yes, your cell phone. Ideally, I would have you minimize all screen use an hour before bed (around the same time I've suggested you dim the lighting around you), but I understand how getting someone to minimize their screen time can often be an impossible ask.

A lot of people I know justify being on their phones before bed to unwind, but they're actually ramping up instead. The glow from TVs, cell phones, and tablets not only suppresses melatonin, it also puts your brain on alert by stimulating photoreceptors that sense light and dark within the retinas of your eyes. Keeping that in mind, I highly recommend blue-light-blocking glasses from WHOOP. You should use these an hour or so before bedtime for better sleep.

Eat nothing heavy. In a perfect world, I would encourage you not to eat two to three hours before going to bed—but sometimes that's not always possible. For example, if you work the late shift, you may not be able to put off eating, and going to bed hungry can be just as disruptive to your sleep. But if you do have to eat something, don't eat at least thirty minutes before bedtime and make sure that it's nothing too heavy.

I'm not suggesting this because the body tends to store more calories as body fat at nighttime. It's because the process of digestion itself can negatively impact your quality of sleep. The heavier the meal, the more insulin your body is forced to release, which can alter your body's circadian rhythm. That's why if you must have something, light, bland foods are best.

At bedtime

Take 250 to 400 milligrams of magnesium bisglycinate. To help my clients recover, I recommend they take this super supplement before going to sleep, as well as after games, performances, hard practices, and intense exercise sessions.

The reason? Not only does magnesium support a better night's sleep, but it also reduces inflammation and boosts athletic performance. It's even considered an immune system booster since T-cells require a decent amount of magnesium to operate efficiently and eradicate abnormal and infected cells within your body.[8] However, the reason I prefer magnesium bisglycinate (a combination of magnesium and the amino acid glycine) is that I've found straight magnesium can sometimes decrease appetite and/or cause diarrhea in some individuals.

How much to take depends—the harder you've trained that day, the more your body needs to help relax your muscles and improve sleep. Initially, start with 250 milligrams, but know there really isn't a downside to taking a higher dose if your digestive system can handle it.

Drink 6 to 8 ounces of tart cherry juice. The bitterness is worth the benefits, which include a faster recovery time when it comes to your strength, as well as a reduction in blood pressure,[9] inflammation, and oxidative stress,[10] which can occur from strenuous physical activity.

Make the room completely dark. I've always been a believer in sleeping in complete darkness, and now science is starting to understand why. Research out of the Center for Circadian and Sleep Medicine at Northwestern University Feinberg School of Medicine[11] discovered that sleeping with a dim light—picture a television with the sound off—for just *one* night impaired subjects' cardiovascular and glucose regulation (fancy speak for having raised heart rate and blood sugar levels), both risk factors for metabolic syndrome, heart disease, and diabetes.

If there's light you can't turn off for any reason—an outside streetlight, for example, or your partner stays up longer than you do on their phones—then invest in blackout shades or an eye mask to minimize exposure to light.

FINALLY, SOMETHING I'M OFTEN ASKED about is melatonin, a hormone supplement popular among some people to assist with sleeping. Although it's not something I typically recommend because your brain (particularly your pineal gland) naturally produces melatonin—a hormone that helps regulate the body's sleep cycle—I don't have a problem with others exploring it if they wish because research has shown it to be nonaddictive and safe. In fact, melatonin has been proven to have other recuperative properties that help your body mend, including lowering cortisol and promoting cellular regeneration by raising HGH (human growth hormone). However, like I said, it's still something that your body already makes on its own, and using some of the suggestions I've already offered (such as minimizing screen time before bed, performing my mobility regimen early in the day, and sleeping in a dark room) will help your body naturally boost the release of this sleep-inducing hormone.

Soothe Your Muscles and/or Mind with at Least One Form of Recuperative Therapy

Everybody knows the concept of fight or flight, when you are forced to make a choice under stress: Do I take on this obstacle in front of me, or do I run as far away as possible from it? Whatever decision you make, whether you choose to start throwing fists or make a mad dash in the exact opposite direction of trouble, it takes energy—and that's energy your body has to quickly pull together from other places.

It does so by immediately releasing both adrenaline and cortisol, a stress hormone secreted by the adrenal glands that elevates your blood sugar and blood pressure. The two let you tap into excess energy, but when that happens, your body sort of shuts down what it doesn't consider top priority in the presence of immediate danger, including your sex drive, digestion, and, unfortunately, your immune system.

Constant stress keeps you in a perpetual state of fight or flight. Your body doesn't understand that the business proposal you're freaking out about isn't a saber-tooth tiger. Your body doesn't get that having to juggle five kids' activities on the same day isn't a life-threatening situation. It just reacts in the way it has for as long as mankind has existed, keeping your cortisol levels elevated so you have plenty of energy—at the expense of your immune system.

In the short term, too much cortisol causes a flood of problems, including fatigue, high blood pressure, low libido, cravings for sugary and fatty food, insomnia, chronic pain, headaches, and an inability to think and concentrate—and that's just the tip of the iceberg. If left unchecked, high cortisol levels due to stress have been shown to contribute to depression, ulcers, digestive problems, chronic back pain, blood clotting and elevated blood cholesterol, arthritis, heart disease, weight gain, and, yes, premature aging.

The good news is you can minimize your body's response to stress (that release of cortisol) for the most part. However, waiting until you're stressed out before doing something about it is sort of like brushing your teeth *after* you find out you have a cavity. That's why I prefer a preemptive strike. You want to attack stress before it attacks you because the longer you let things linger—the longer you put off things in the now—the more time stress has to break you down.

You'll already have recognized and addressed in the Eat portion of the book a few of the things that could be stressing you out. But there are other ways you can help your mind and body heal at the highest level. Capitalizing on these "mending moments" will boost your immune system, elevate your mood, relax your muscles, relieve pain, and activate your parasympathetic nervous system—your body's "rest and digest" mode—speeding recovery. All it takes is trying to fit at least one of these mending moments into your day, each and every day.

Get a Massage

We're all familiar with having a "cheat meal" once a week, when we splurge and allow ourselves to eat whatever we want. Consider this your "treat meal"—a treatment that may feel indulgent, but it's extremely important for recovery and longevity.

Typically, people wait until they ache all over before they consider getting a massage, but most athletes don't because their jobs depend on their ability to perform. Instead, they lock in regular massages to head off possible problems at the pass so that pain and discomfort never sideline them later. They keep themselves loose and relaxed before their muscles can even think about tensing up in the first place. But most important, they know the benefits of massage go far beyond just feeling good.

Besides improving blood circulation and alleviating muscle soreness,[12] according to data out of the Buck Institute for Research on Aging, massages not only improve range of motion and reduce inflammation, but encourage the growth of new mitochondria in skeletal muscle on a cellular level.[13] That means a massage can help your muscles heal stronger and faster after exercise or activity.

From a mentally therapeutic perspective, it should always be done by someone who's skilled and trusted, if you have the means and ability to do so. That said, I entirely understand the amount of time, money, and commitment that requires, but there are plenty of other more convenient, less-pricey options at your disposal. You could strike a deal with a spouse, partner, or close friend, contact a local massage therapy school to see if it offers free or reduced-rates from students in training, or even check with your doctor to see if you have any conditions (such as stress-related issues or anxiety) that warrant regular massages that could be covered by insurance.

If none of the above suggestions are possible for you, then your next best option is to do it yourself. Although I'm not big on self-massage, you can still loosen up your muscles and release any knots by investing in either a foam roller or a therapeutic massage gun, like the Hyperice Hypervolt or Vyper. Presently, these two pieces of equipment are the most cost-effective devices to therapeutically massage soft tissues (your muscles, connective tissue, tendons, and ligaments) in a safe and easy way.

Meditate

I highly believe in meditation and don't prefer one technique over the other. Whether you prefer movement meditation (such as tai chi or yoga), visualization (which has you picture a certain image in your mind), progressive (where you contract and relax one muscle group at a time), or mantra meditation (a technique that has you focus on a particular word, sound, or mantra), there isn't really any right or wrong way. So long as you connect with the technique and it relaxes you, then I encourage you to stick with it.

However, I do lean more toward mindfulness meditation because of the abundant research that's been done on its effects and how simple it is. It's not over-the-top spiritual, and instead it requires nothing more than having you focus on deep breathing and noticing the thoughts that float into your brain.

Proven to both reduce chronic pain[14] and drastically lower blood-based markers associated with stress, including the adrenocorticotropic hormone (ACTH) as well as inflammatory proteins, this technique has been shown to significantly improve energy levels, brain function,[15] and decision-making.[16] The problem is this type of meditation can have the exact opposite effect if you don't know how to do it properly:

- If possible, change into loose, comfortable clothing so you won't be distracted.
- Find a quiet spot where you won't be bothered.
- Sit naturally. There's no specific posture you have to assume—just position yourself any way that feels relaxing to you. You should, however, be seated upright so that you don't fall asleep.
- Consider setting a timer. You don't necessarily have to, but if it keeps you from being distracted by constantly wondering how long you've been meditating then use it.
- Start by taking nice, deep breaths and focus on how your belly and lungs rise and fall.
- As thoughts come into your head, acknowledge them—don't try to ignore them—then imagine they're just passing by like clouds.
- Stick with it for five minutes to start, even if you feel like you can do more. Then begin to add more time to your meditations as you become more comfortable with them until you're able to carve out a space of between twenty to thirty minutes.

Last point: Don't beat yourself up if you don't remain completely in the moment every time. Instead of clearing their minds, some people make the mistake of using the time to think of their to-do lists. Remember that, in most cases, there's nothing you can knock off that list in that moment. But what will help you tackle it is having more energy, feeling less stressed overall, and boosting your focus—all of which you'll experience afterward if you allow yourself to meditate properly.

Ice Up!

First and foremost, let me start by saying if you're dealing with an actual injury, then it's more important to see your doctor than grab ice out of your freezer. I say this because most people tend to "ice up" only when they need to bring swelling down from an injury. But if you're not hurt and just experiencing the usual soreness that comes with being active, ice can be hugely helpful.

The magic of ice is in how it quickly contracts your blood vessels, minimizing inflammation within your muscles and joints, which can speed up recovery,[17] especially after a high-performance day. You can incorporate it in a few different ways:

Take a soak. Ice baths (also known as cold water immersion) are definitely hardcore, but they're easy enough to safely pull off at home:

- Fill your tub about a third of the way with cold water.
- Add a layer of ice—shoot for a ratio of about 3:1 water to ice. (Fortunately ice floats, so if you're not sure of the ratio, you can eyeball it with a ruler.)
- Check your temperature—use a pool or meat thermometer to make sure that it's not too cold. The sweet spot is between 50 to 60°F.
- Now for the hardest part—getting in! Slowly ease into the tub, making sure that you're completely covering any parts that feel inflamed.
- Stick it out for at least ten minutes, but no longer than fifteen.

Grab a bag. It doesn't take much to ice down your knees, ankles, back, and other crucial areas once or twice a day. I like Hyperice's products because of how they conform and stay put on certain areas that can be difficult to ice, such as the shoulders and lower back. But if you don't have any fancy stuff available or need to do it on the cheap:

- Grab a medium to large Ziploc bag and fill it halfway with ice.
- Place a very thin washcloth or hand towel over the area you'll be icing (to prevent direct contact between your skin and the bag), then place the bag onto the area.
- Wrap an Ace bandage around the bag (not too tight, but just enough to keep the ice from shifting).
- Leave the bag on the area for ten to fifteen minutes tops.
- Repeat the process with a new bag on any other problem areas.

Find a bucket. I'm not talking about doing the ice bucket challenge here. What I suggest to clients is even if they've had a day in which they haven't done much physically, icing down your ankles and feet is still something you can do anytime. Not only will you be giving some attention to one of the most-neglected parts of your body, you'll also cool down and rejuvenate your whole body. Here's the best way to do it:

- Put down a heavy beach towel (to absorb any potential spillover, plus to give yourself something to dry your feet on afterward).
- Grab a thick Rubbermaid bucket and fill a third of it with ice.
- Pour cold water into the bucket.
- Put your feet into the bucket and shimmy them down until your soles touch the bottom.
- Keep your feet in the bucket for ten to fifteen minutes maximum.

You might think that doing this at the end of the day is best, but there honestly isn't a bad time to do it. In fact, if you have the opportunity, give it a shot at different times and see how you feel, both immediately afterward and a few hours later.

Warm (never hot!) Epsom salt baths. I use these with LeBron the night before big games for maybe twenty to thirty minutes tops. I never do it on game day because it takes some time to rehydrate your muscles prior to the game. But when we do it the night before, that soak does a fantastic job of relaxing his muscles and relieving both stress and pain.

Could you do the same thing the day before a high-performance day, specifically one that will challenge you physically? Absolutely, but if you don't want to interfere with your sleep, here's the proper order of things to do if you have the time:

- Take an Epsom salt bath in the early evening, roughly an hour before bedtime. I recommend pouring in about a cup of Epsom salt, and making sure the water is just warm enough to help melt the salt crystals, but no hotter than that.

- After twenty to thirty minutes, step out, drain the tub, then get back in and take a quick cold shower to both rinse off and lower your internal temperature. By the time you're finished, you should be about thirty minutes away from bedtime.

Take a Few Deep Breaths at Least Once Every Hour

Yes, taking a few deep breaths helps lower your blood pressure, delivers more energy-rich oxygen throughout your body, and stimulates the parasympathetic nervous system—all great reasons to do it every hour. But the benefits of slow, concentrated breathing go far beyond stress relief and healing.

Recent research has proven that deep, controlled breathing at a slow pace significantly reduces feelings of pain, optimizes how your brain cognitively processes things including perception and emotion,[18] and may even increase your attention span by releasing noradrenaline, a chemical messenger in the brain.[19] By doing this every hour, you're not only reaping all these amazing benefits, but it's also naturally making you more mindful of how you're breathing in between those hours—and that's my goal.

My hope is that, by practicing deep breathing every hour, you'll unconsciously begin to breathe more deeply and into your diaphragm (not your chest) all day long—so that you experience all these longevity-enhancing benefits 24/7. But even if that takes time to lock in, you'll still experience all the advantages that come from simply allowing yourself to breathe a little better at different points throughout the day.

The rules are simple—set a timer on your phone for sixty minutes, then when it goes off, no matter where you are, here's what I expect you to do:

- Start with your mouth closed and slowly inhale through your nose (as deeply as you can) for a count of four seconds. I want you to focus on filling your belly (not your chest) with as much air as possible. I want your stomach to extend out and away from your body—do not let feeling fat or bloated get in the way.
- Hold your breath for a count of four seconds.
- Slowly exhale either out of your nose or mouth for a count of four seconds.
- Pause for four seconds.
- Repeat the four steps at least four times.

This 4–4–4–4 pattern (inhale for four seconds, hold for four seconds, exhale for four seconds, pause for four seconds) is called box breathing and is typically my go-to. However, another technique that's equally effective is a variation of box breathing that I like to call the "4–2–8–2," which changes things a bit like so:

- Breathe through your nose for a count of four. Try to completely fill and expand your belly as far as possible.
- Hold your breath for a count of two.
- Slowly exhale out of your mouth with your lips pursed (like you're blowing out a candle) for a count of eight—if you can go even slower, have at it! Ideally, you should exhale as much as you can until your lungs feel empty.
- Pause for two seconds.
- Repeat the four steps six to eight times.

Whether you choose the 4–4–4–4 or 4–2–8–2 pattern, it doesn't have to be precise. Ideally, since you're probably using your phone to alert yourself every hour, using the timer to track how many seconds you're inhaling, exhaling, and holding is a great option. However, if you're anyplace where you may feel self-conscious, just count in your head as best as possible. So long as you're going as slowly as possible, you'll still reap the same benefits.

You're finished! Who would've ever thought that getting the body to relax would require so much effort, am I right? But remember, that's the thing: The reason why so many people suffer from not being in an optimal state of healing is because they assume that just *doing nothing* gives their body time to heal. You're no longer a part of that club—now let's break down everything you did.

CHAPTER 13

Break It Down

After every game and every workout session, I sit with LeBron and walk through how his body feels. Muscle, joint, and mind, we explore how every part of him is doing so that we can assess what he needs in recovery. We look for areas that seem tighter than usual and sorer than before but spend just as much attention recognizing the areas that feel fresh and ready to go again. Because recovery isn't about only focusing on what aches—it's also figuring out why other parts of you don't. Every piece of your body is interconnected, and looking for those networks can take your recovery to a whole different stratosphere.

1: How Do You Feel Now Compared to Then?

By now, you know the drill. It's time to reflect on the assessments I asked you to take in Chapter 11, starting with sleep:

As soon as you wake up. I want you to reflect on the same four things I asked you to reflect on an hour before bedtime:

1. How hard did you push yourself physically today?
2. How hard did you push yourself mentally today?
3. Where would you rank your stress level?
4. How tired do you feel right now?

The first two I'll address in a moment because what's most important is addressing how you feel after a full night's rest.

Stress level: Obviously, the lower this number is, the better your chances of deep, sound sleep. But if that number is higher than it was the night before, I want you to consider why. Because right now, you're already beginning to stress out for some reason, most likely regarding how the rest of your day is about to go. Question is, can you do something about it today so that you wake up less stressed tomorrow? For example, maybe you're stressed because:

- You woke up late. (If that's the case, then make sure that doesn't happen tomorrow.)
- You're about to have a really chaotic day. (If that's it, could you have planned for it? If so, strategize better the next time.)
- You have a problem that's not instantly fixable. (I get that certain life situations are out of our control, but is there a way to improve that situation or minimize—even a little bit—how that situation is affecting you?)

My point is, first thing in the morning, you don't necessarily know all the twists and turns that might come out of left field that day—the obstacles that can quickly turn a bad morning into an even worse afternoon. That means the only things that should be on your mind (and causing you stress) are things you're aware of, situations within your immediate view and problems you could potentially do something about.

Here's the problem with that: If you're waking up stressed, your brain isn't just thinking about those problems in that moment—it was most likely worrying about those same problems as you slept. And even if those stressors didn't prevent you from falling asleep normally, they could still be disrupting your circadian rhythm and potentially reducing your time spent in REM sleep.

That's why I want you to seriously reflect on these two sets of numbers (both before bedtime and upon waking up) and remind yourself that what's concerning you before you sleep could be deteriorating your quality of sleep. Try to get those numbers to drop by taking control of those stressors during the day.

Tiredness: Obviously, the ideal number is 1—if not 0. Not being tired is the entire point of sleep! But if that number is higher for any reason—and it's a problem that seems to be consistent—then it's a clear indicator that certain changes need to be made, all of which I'll address in the next chapter.

How hard you pushed yourself physically and mentally. I ask you to consider these numbers for a few reasons:

- **It points out temporary problems.** Having a day in which you went full steam at your job, trimmed trees in your backyard, coached your kid's back-to-back soccer games—any day when it's obvious you were far more active than usual—can leave your body still feeling exhausted the next day, despite getting seven to eight perfect hours of quality sleep. In cases like this, I don't want you to beat yourself up thinking you did anything wrong if you wake up feeling wrecked.
- **It points out hidden problems.** On the other hand, if you did nothing difficult physically or mentally the day before but still woke up not feeling refreshed after seven to eight hours, it's an indicator that something is off, which means I really want you to seriously reflect on some of the suggestions I'm about to make.

After trying other tactics from Chapter 12—I also asked you to consider the following right before taking a few deep breaths each hour, as well as before whatever recuperative therapy you may have used to soothe your muscles/mind (massage, meditation, icing, a warm Epsom salt bath):

- Where would you rank your energy level?
- How calm do you feel right now?
- How would you rank how achy/sore/tight you feel overall (head to toe)?

Energy and calm levels: How this number should change really depends on you. Any of the interventions above might leave you feeling more energized, calmer, and more tranquil (which you could interpret as less energy) or be difficult to gauge. There is no wrong answer—all the above are perfectly fine—but I just want you to note any differences so that you make a stronger connection with the effectiveness of each tactic on both your energy and well-being.

Achy/sore/tight: Even though doing a head-to-toe "pain check" typically doesn't apply to deep breathing, I want you to gauge how you honestly feel now after whichever recuperative therapy you chose. The truth is, some therapies work better than others for different people, but in any case, this number should drop to some degree. If it doesn't, then you may need to consider whether you are following the techniques correctly.

2. What Took It to the Next Level?

The mending motivators I swear by may require less effort compared to watching your diet or following my mobility program daily, but that doesn't mean there aren't circumstances that might have made them easier to accomplish.

Atmosphere: Even though my mending motivators may differ from one another, they all require you to feel comfortable—and your surroundings play a huge part in that. You can't sleep as soundly, breathe as deeply, or allow your body to completely relax if you're not content in the space you're in. Consider the surroundings when you felt your best to determine if there was anything particular around you that put you more at ease.

Preparation: You might think these tactics—sleeping, meditating, getting a massage—don't require much prep, but they do. And if having everything you needed at the ready helped make things less stressful and easier to pull off, whether it was making sure you had comfortable clothes to meditate or sleep in, or plenty of prepared ice in the freezer—then give those helping hands their due and try to make them a habit for next time.

Acceptance: It can be difficult for a lot of people to take these mending motivators seriously because of what feels to be less effort required. But if that wasn't you—if one reason you benefited more was because you completely embraced how these tactics are just as important as diet and exercise when it comes to longevity—then I want you to not only stay in that place mentally but apply it to the other tactics as well.

3. What Stood in the Way of Success?

Like I said before, my mending motivators—the simple tactics that go a long way in helping your body heal itself—don't require much effort, but they do require your participation. So if you're not able to do any of them on a regular basis, then you need to reflect on what or who might be keeping you from enjoying the longevity you deserve.

Outside opinion: I'm not going to lie—some people might look at what you're about to do as decadent, questionable, or lame. Was the reason you didn't pause to breathe deeply for a minute because your coworkers or friends were around you at that moment? Did you avoid going to bed at a decent hour because you didn't want to be the first one saying good night in your family? Are you nervous about what others might think if they find out you're booking a massage every week?

Is that you? If being concerned about what others think of your actions is holding you back in any way from doing them as effectively or in the right amount of time—or worse, from doing them at all—then blame me. I'm serious. Pull out this book and point to every reason why I'm asking you to do these things. None of these tactics are ineffective or self-indulgent. Instead, what they are collectively is a series of basic, proven techniques that improve and extend not just health and productivity—but *your* health and productivity. None of your "rocks" should object to them, and if they do, then it might be time to question the company you keep.

Distraction: Did a noisy environment make it impossible to meditate or sleep? Was your day so chaotic that you lost track of time and forgot to set up some form of therapy or you didn't bother to breathe every hour?

Is that you? The good news: These types of distractions are preventable with better planning. My high performers are pulled in hundreds of directions every day on top of experiencing unfamiliarity and distraction at every turn when traveling. And yet they still find time for these tactics because they understand the health, mobility, and longevity benefits that come from them. They don't *hope* that nothing sidetracks them—they acknowledge present and potential problems so they can quickly turn any obstacle into an afterthought.

Misplaced priorities: To heal faster and more efficiently, you must put recovery—you must put *yourself*—at the top of your priority list. But sometimes that's easier said than done because of how selfish some of these tactics might feel to you. Other times, you may inadvertently be doing things you "believe" put yourself first but are actually causing you to land in last place.

Is that you? We all do things every day that technically don't add value to our lives—and that's fine. Sometimes we need to binge-watch that show, mindlessly scroll through a news feed, or do something that seemingly doesn't benefit us, motivate us, or move the needle in any way—but those moments still serve a purpose. It becomes a problem when you let too many of those moments occur to the point where your entire day is filled up with activities that have little to no value.

From this point on, you need to make yourself priority number one and not feel a single ounce of guilt about it. You need to reflect on all of the ways you're "treating" yourself throughout the day and question the value of each. Simply put, when considering whatever is preventing you from prioritizing these tactics in your day, you need to question if it's "healing you forward" or holding you back.

CHAPTER 14

Rebuild It Better

Congratulations, you made it to the final portion of the book. But just because the mending motivators you've incorporated into your life have you well on your way to shifting the healing process into overdrive, that doesn't mean you're done. In fact, there are plenty of things to pay attention to that can impact your recovery, both positively and negatively. In this last chapter, it's time to reconsider and retweak a few aspects of your daily routine to maximize your mending.

Are You Overtraining?

Some people have a hard time understanding that just because something's good for you doesn't mean more is better. If you push yourself too hard, you can overtax your central nervous system and prevent your body from proper healing and recovery. In particular, overtraining comes with some not-so-fun symptoms, such as:

- a loss of appetite or other digestive issues
- constant joint pain (and/or muscle soreness)
- a gradual and/or sharp drop in performance
- an increase in infections, injuries, or colds
- restlessness and/or difficulty falling asleep
- chronic fatigue (despite getting enough sleep)
- feelings of anxiety, depression, and/or moodiness

These signs of overtraining are your body telling you to pull back the reins. Two things, right off the bat:

1. My mobility routine is designed to be used every day and should never lead to overtraining. But it's those extracurricular activities you may be doing that I can't see—those marathon workouts or pushing yourself too hard physically in your job, sport, yardwork, whatever the case may be—that could be preventing your body from healing as efficiently as it should.

   Ironically, my mobility program sometimes leads to overtraining because it opens new doors. Clients notice such a drastic improvement in their performance that they strive for higher levels of physical activity that they didn't think would ever be within their reach—and I'm all for it. The trick is making sure you're not pushing yourself so hard that you can't recover quickly enough, because everybody has a limit.
2. Give it a week. If you've only been doing a new activity for a few days, your symptoms are unlikely to be overtraining. It's actually natural to sometimes experience what feels like overtraining when putting your body through paces it's not used to, perhaps because you have been inactive for a while, are using a new lifting plan, or are playing a sport you've never played before. But if you're still feeling those ill effects after week one, that's when you must look at whether you're pushing your body too far.

So, **how can you keep it from happening in the first place?** The good news is that some of the more common causes of overtraining are issues my program should help you avoid: poor nutrition, stress, and lack of sleep. However, you might still be at risk of pushing both your muscles and central nervous system too hard in other ways. The best way to prevent that—and keep your body in a constant state of mending—is to strive for moderation:

Be cautious if you're going over 300 minutes' worth. Science is clear that engaging in regular moderate physical activity between 150 to 300 minutes weekly is tremendous in lowering your risk of pretty much every medical condition you can think of, from diabetes, cancer, cardiovascular disease, and obesity.[1] But past the 300-minute mark, the health returns are minimal,[2] so unless you're participating in a sport or activity that demands that sort of training, you might not want to push past that boundary.

Sidenote: You might think that walking 10,000 steps daily could easily push you past 300 minutes—and you wouldn't be wrong. However, done in the traditional sense (meaning, walking at a normal pace on mostly flat surfaces like we usually walk around during the day), 10,000 steps is typically considered a low-intensity form of exercise that shouldn't lead to overtraining.

Give yourself enough recovery time. Take off at least one day (and preferably two) each week, avoiding exercise or any moderate-intensity activity. If you're regularly doing a weight-training routine, then never train a muscle group intensely more than twice a week. Ideally, you want to allow each muscle group to rest from between forty-eight to seventy-two hours, particularly after any intense, heavy resistance training.

When in doubt, take your pulse before breakfast. Everybody's body is different, so what could cause you to experience overtraining symptoms might not have any effect on someone else. However, no matter what your body's tolerance for training is, there's a fast way to figure out whether you're pushing your body too hard or too much.

Before you begin doing any new routine, make a practice of taking your pulse first thing in the morning as soon as you get out of bed. Write down that number, then continue checking your pulse every morning, especially the morning after a high-performance day. If it's ever higher than eight or more beats per minute above that base number you originally wrote down, give your body a rest day to refresh itself and recuperate.

Here's what's going on: The fitter you are, the lower your resting heart rate generally becomes as your cardiovascular health improves. However, on days you overexert yourself with exercise or activity, your resting blood pressure elevates naturally as a result but quickly stabilizes to its normal level soon afterward. It's a reaction to that stress you've placed on yourself and it's entirely normal. However, when you push yourself too far and don't give your body enough time to recover, your resting blood pressure never gets the chance to stabilize and stays at a raised rate for a longer period. It stays in that reactive *elevated* state that isn't healthy, but it's a great way to know if you need a break—if you listen to what your body is trying to tell you.

Never Say No to Naps

Obviously, there is no algorithm for LeBron. When the whole world is watching you perform—when you need to be at your very best when everyone else is a few hours away from heading to bed—you can't leave anything to chance. LeBron's pregame routine often starts at 6:00 or 7:00 p.m. at the earliest. That leaves time for an afternoon nap if it's needed.

There isn't any specific amount of time he'll shoot for. Instead, he wisely listens to his body's requirements for additional sleep (beyond what he gets each evening). He might nap twenty minutes one day and two hours the next, depending on where he's at in his schedule and how hard he's pushed himself. He's learned, from long experience, *what* his body needs and *when* it needs it.

Now, when it comes to other clients—and when it comes to you—I recommend a variation of this strategy because LeBron's body and the demands he puts on it are entirely different from the average person's. Instead, I recommend (when needed) to take a nap between ten and thirty minutes max—ideally right after lunch. Not only will you feel more refreshed the rest of the day, but research has shown that short naps are effective at relieving stress and bolstering the immune system,[3] significantly improving memory,[4] and even slowing down how fast your brain shrinks as you age.[5]

A couple easy ground rules to follow:

- Don't go over thirty minutes—any longer and you run the risk of having more difficulty falling asleep that evening. If you're still tired afterward, splash some cold water on your face to help shake off the grogginess.
- Try not to nap after 2:00 p.m.—that's the cut-off point most sleep experts agree on. Any later in the day could affect your ability to experience enough REM sleep later that night.

Amplify It All

Amplify Your Sleep

Add some weight. One thing that I really enjoy is using a weighted blanket because of its calming effect. They actually mimic a form of deep-touch therapy (sort of like a swaddled infant) that eases anxiety and helps you fall asleep faster. In fact, research has shown that subjects suffering from insomnia experienced reduced insomnia severity, improved sleep, and less daytime sleepiness when using them.[6] Don't want to invest in one just yet? Then make a cheaper version by layering some extra blankets on top of you.

Change your sheets! And not just because your mom told you to. You should change them especially often if you find yourself waking up sweaty. Ideally, you want to sleep in breathable materials (such as Coolmax, bamboo, natural linen, polyester, or cotton) that help wick sweat away from your skin—and wash the sheets often. According to the National Sleep Foundation, about three out of four people say they've experienced a more comfortable sleep when their sheets smelled fresh and clean.

Cool yourself down in other ways. If you can't drop the temperature when sleeping or just want to try a different way to chill, experiment with a few other options such as cooling pillows, bedding, or mattress pads. Or try a few cheaper DIY options, such as:

- putting your pillowcases in the freezer
- turning on a fan (even in wintertime)
- drinking ice-cold water before bed
- placing an ice pack behind your neck

Plan ahead, but not in bed. Thinking about what you need to accomplish the next day while lying in bed only leaves you worrying about things you need to do while you're in no position to get them done, which can make it harder to fall asleep. Instead, make a conscious effort to run through tomorrow's to-do list two hours *before* going to sleep. Doing this may still bring on stress in that moment, but you'll be in a better position to think things through—or possibly even tackle a "tomorrow task" that evening so that it's off your mind by the time you climb under the sheets.

Avoid nicotine and alcohol. Some people get the impression that these vices help them relax, but what they both do not only causes you to have trouble falling and staying asleep, but negatively suppresses REM sleep, allowing you to experience less deep sleep—and less healing as a result.

Stick with a schedule. Behind the scenes, your body relies on a circadian biological clock that regulates how tired or alert you feel over the course of twenty-four hours. It's great at its job when left to do it, but when you're erratic with what time you head to bed throughout the week, it disrupts your natural sleep cycle. To keep that internal clock running smoothly (and help you experience more REM sleep), the trick is to stick with a time not just on weekdays, but weekends as well when you might be more tempted to go to bed later and linger in bed longer the next day.

Because all my clients cross time zones on a regular basis—yet are still expected to perform at the absolute best, no matter how disrupted their sleep cycles might be as a result—I'm often asked if there's a trick that quickly stabilizes their circadian rhythm that goes beyond naps and minimizing light during the evening. But the easiest and most effective solution I always suggest is to simply prepare ahead.

All my clients know where on Earth (and what time zone) they're going to find themselves on their schedules well ahead of time, which is why I advise them to prepare for each time zone *days before* they find themselves *in* that time zone, if possible. Meaning, if they know they're going to be flying someplace two or three hours ahead or behind their present time (one hour usually isn't that disruptive), then I'll advise them to start adjusting their sleep schedule *one hour each day* a few days prior to match whatever time zone they're traveling to (so long as it doesn't affect things for them in the moment).

For example, if they typically go to bed at ten o'clock and the time difference where they're flying to is going to be two hours ahead (traveling west to east), I'll recommend going to sleep at nine o'clock (and waking up an hour earlier) starting one or two days before they fly. If the time difference is two hours behind (traveling east to west), I'll suggest hitting the sack around eleven o'clock and waking up an hour later in the morning. The same rules apply if it's a three-hour time difference, but I just have them start the process two or three days before traveling, adjusting the time they go to bed (and wake up) by one hour the first day, then by two hours the second day.

Is this trick always doable or foolproof for my clientele? Not always, especially because of how intense their schedule is from city to city. But for most people, prepping yourself a few days prior can keep your circadian rhythm in line so your mending doesn't stop whenever you're on the road.

Amplify Your Restorative Therapies

Mix and match often. As tempting as it might be to stick with the same massage therapist because they did a great job the last time, or only choosing to do meditation over other options I suggested simply because it's easiest, I want you to seriously explore as many possibilities as you can. For example:

- If you've always gotten a deep-tissue massage, venture out and try other forms, such as trigger point, sports, Swedish, hot stone, aromatherapy, reflexology, Thai, or shiatsu, just to mention a few.

- Instead of sticking with one way to ice down, cycle through all the ways before repeating your usual go-to.
- As much as I like mindfulness meditation, challenge yourself to experience as many different forms as possible.

The reason I say this is because even if one form of restorative therapy works wonders for you, each offers a certain number of benefits over others. The more options you experiment with—even if they don't seem as effective as your favorites—the more you'll experience the widest range of benefits that are possible by alternating between different versions.

Get in touch with yourself. There's a technique I sometimes apply to meditation known as progressive muscle relaxation that helps put the body more at ease. The method isn't difficult at all but requires you to flex and relax portions of your body from head to toe.

To do it, either get in a seated position or lie flat on your back. Start by flexing your toes (tight, but not too tight) for at least five or six seconds, then relax for fifteen to twenty seconds, and repeat. From there, travel your way up, applying the same technique to your calves, your thighs, your butt, your lower back, your abdomen, your upper back, your chest, your biceps, your triceps, your forearms, your fingers, your shoulders, then end with your neck.

Amplify Your Breathing

Forget about the one-hour rule. Telling you to perform deep breathing every sixty minutes is far from a hard-and-fast rule. In fact, this is the one technique in this book that you can never overdo, so experiment. Try it every thirty, twenty, or ten minutes if you like, or make a point of doing it every time you sit down, listen to someone, or perform certain tasks. The more often you do it throughout the day, the more often you'll experience its benefits—and the more likely you'll turn it into an unconscious habit.

Do it whenever you feel negative. What do I mean by that? The moment you recognize you're experiencing any negative emotion or feeling—

anxiety, depression, anger, frustration, or self-doubt, for example—any reaction that you feel isn't helping a situation whatsoever, that's when I want you to stop everything and just breathe.

It's not just about how this helps bring about a parasympathetic response that promotes relaxation and recovery, but making a habit of breathing deeply as soon as you recognize you're having a moment forces you to temporarily step back from whatever's triggering that emotion or feeling. Sometimes all it takes is walking away from something momentarily to minimize its effect on your state of mind and allow you to see just how big (or hopefully small) the problem really is.

Shoot to extend those seconds. Even though I gave you two suggestions on how to slow down your breathing—4–4–4–4 or 4–2–8–2—the more often you do it, the more you're going to notice that, if given the opportunity, you could probably slow things down even more. If that's the case, then definitely do so.

These aren't magical numbers. There isn't any specific science attached to inhaling for this number of seconds and exhaling for that number of seconds. They're just numbers that allow you to pay attention to the pace of your breathing so that you can slow it down. But as your lungs and diaphragm become accustomed to drawing in more oxygen-rich air, if you can lengthen those numbers—for example, slowing things down even further to a 5–5–5–5 or 6–6–6–6 pace, or a 5–3–9–3 or 6–4–10–4 tempo—go for it. So long as it feels comfortable to do so, the slower you go, the more benefit you'll be getting from every breath.

Final Thought

Even though you've come to the end of this guide, this isn't the finish line—instead, it's only the beginning of your new journey.

What I want you to remember as you follow my formula is this: if some of the concepts, principles, and methodologies presented ever seem unorthodox and unconventional to you, I ask that you trust this process of mindfulness and accountability for the sake of your health and longevity. I can't speak to what types of programs you've tried in the past, but know that this isn't a collection of tips and tricks randomly put together to fill a book. Every single tactic, tip, and technique serves a greater purpose that builds off each other. And even if you can't connect the dots on how it all comes together for now, you'll see and feel it for yourself soon enough—but only if you stay true to the course I've set for you.

I'll end with this: I've been honored to work with many top performers at the pinnacle of their respective disciplines and they all have the same thing in common. They each started with the simple belief that greatness was possible. Now, it's your turn, and I'm right here to walk this path to greatness with you. Let's go!

Appendix

The 27 Movement Exercises

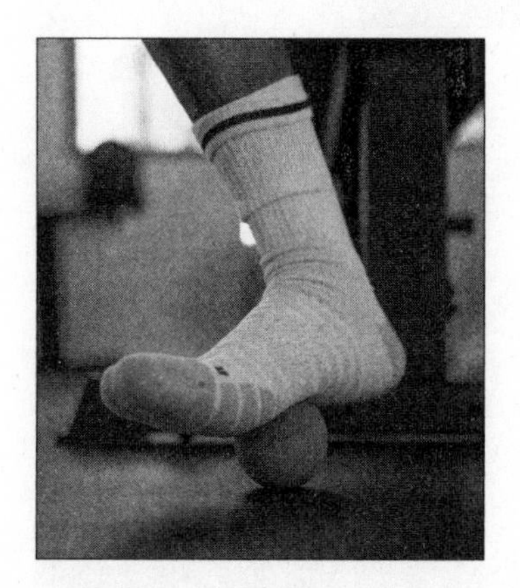

1. Plantar Fascia Stretch

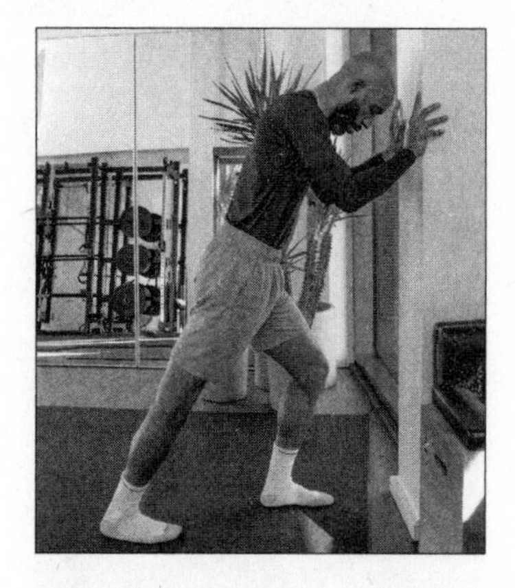

2. Standing Wall Stretch

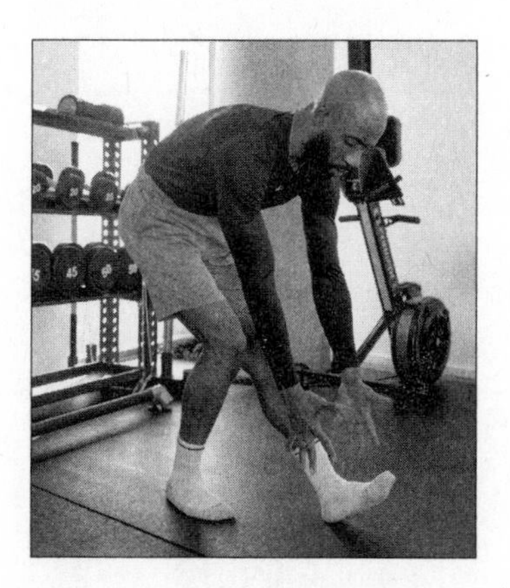

3a. Standing Hamstring and Nerve Floss Stretch

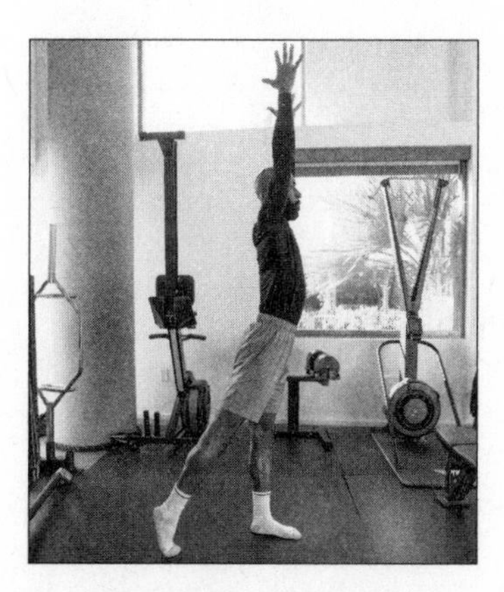

3b. Standing Hamstring and Nerve Floss Stretch

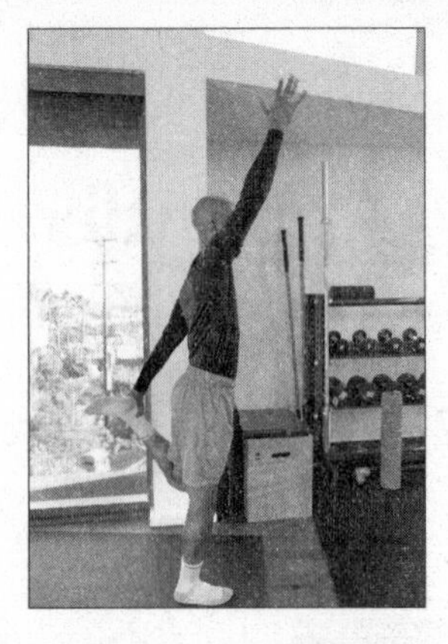

4. Alternating Quad Stretch

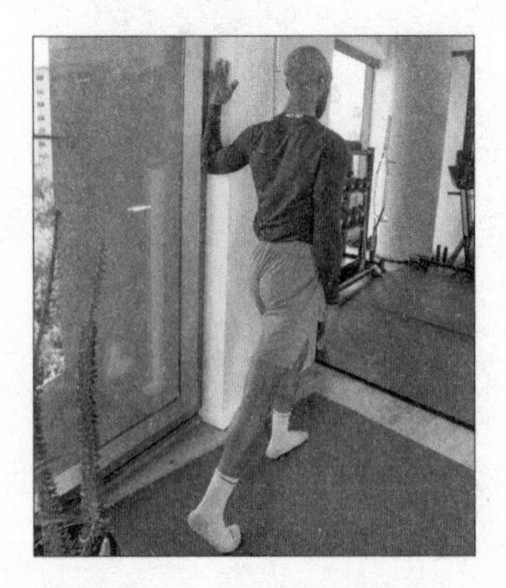

5a. Single-Arm Pectoral Stretch

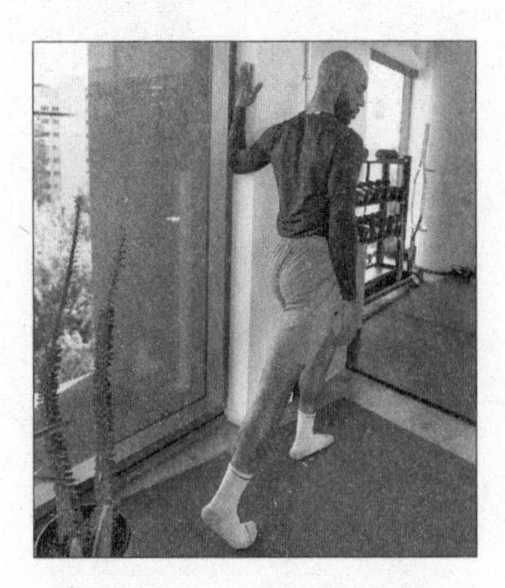

5b. Single-Arm Pectoral Stretch

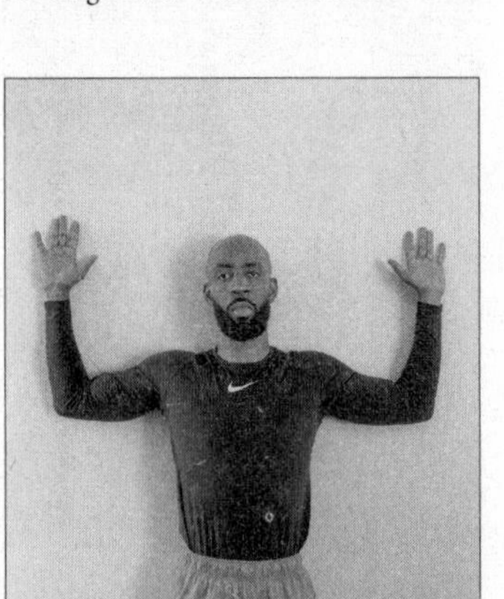

6a. Angel Stretch

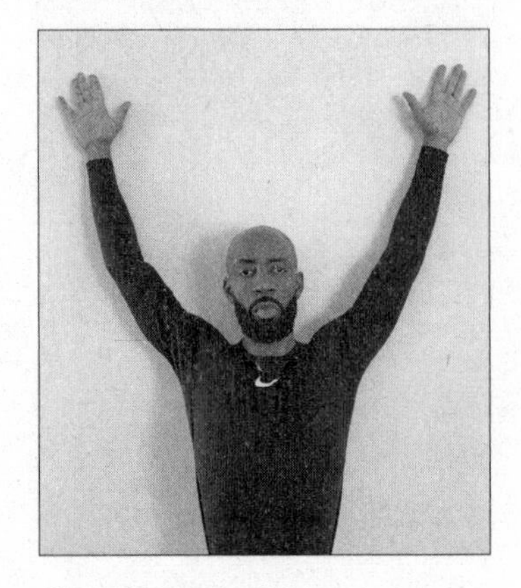

6b. Angel Stretch

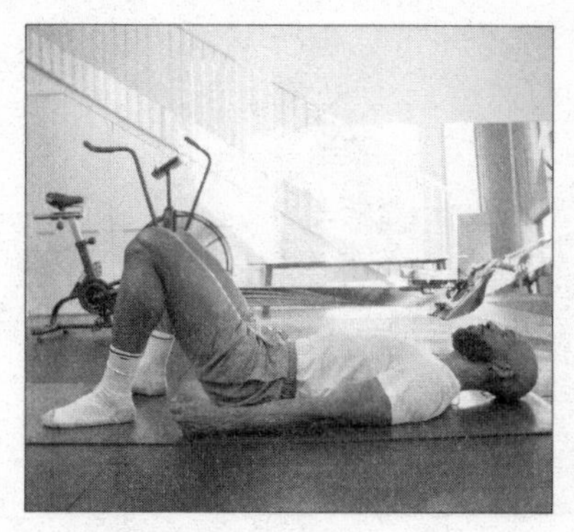

7a. On-the-Floor Marching

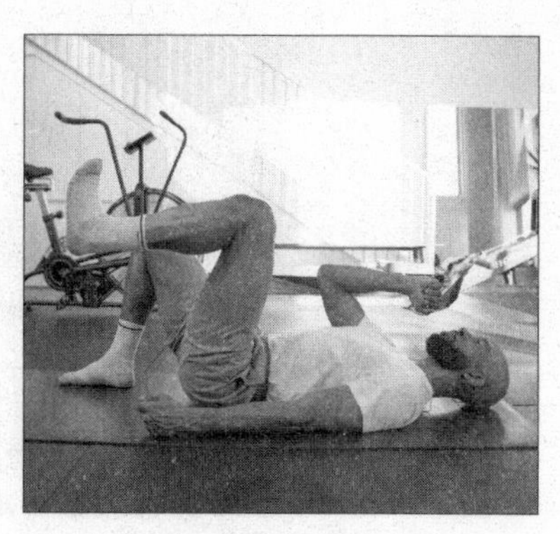

7b. On-the-Floor Marching

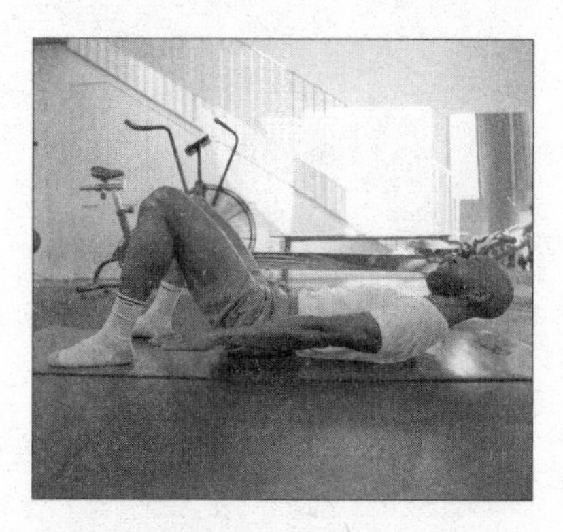

8a. On-the-Floor Pilates 100

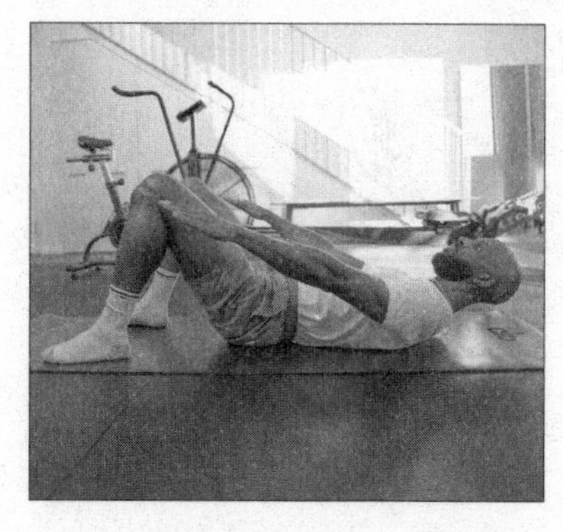

8b. On-the-Floor Pilates 100

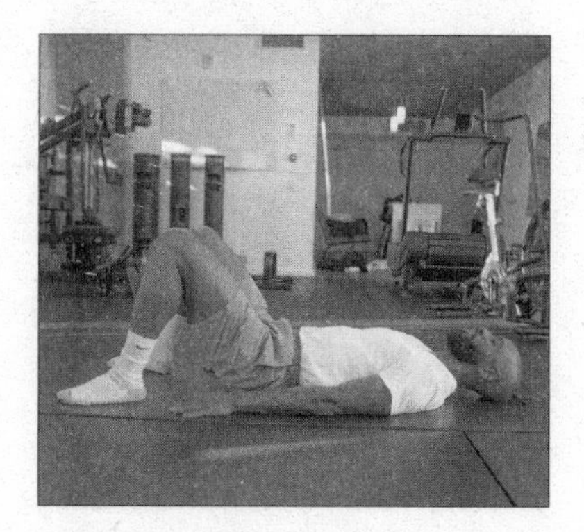

9a. Glute Bridge

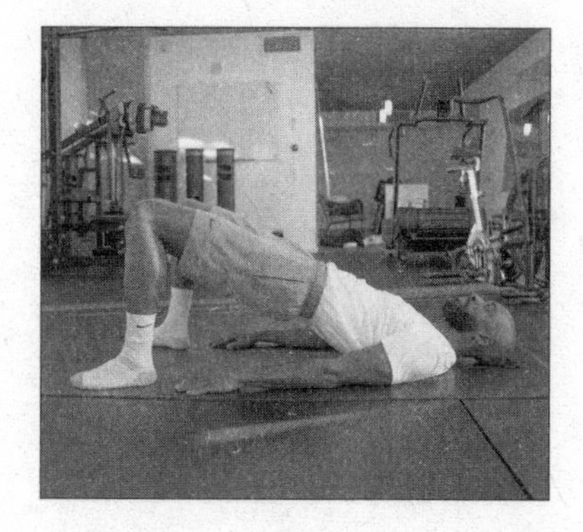

9b. Glute Bridge

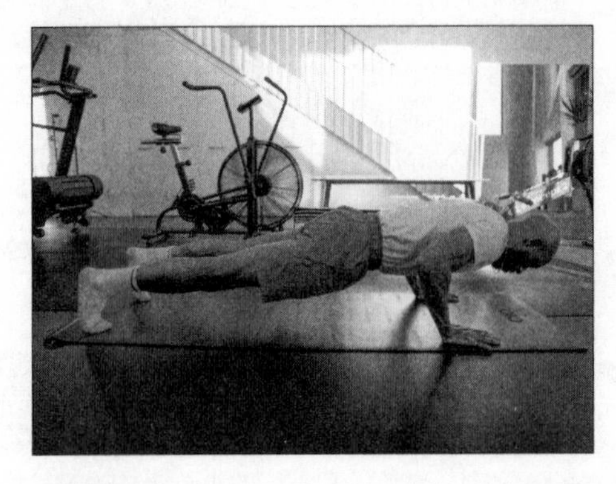

10. Push-Up

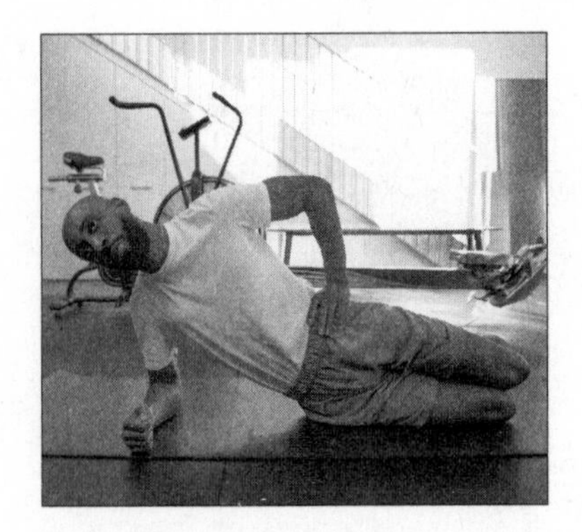

11a. Bent-Knee Side Plank

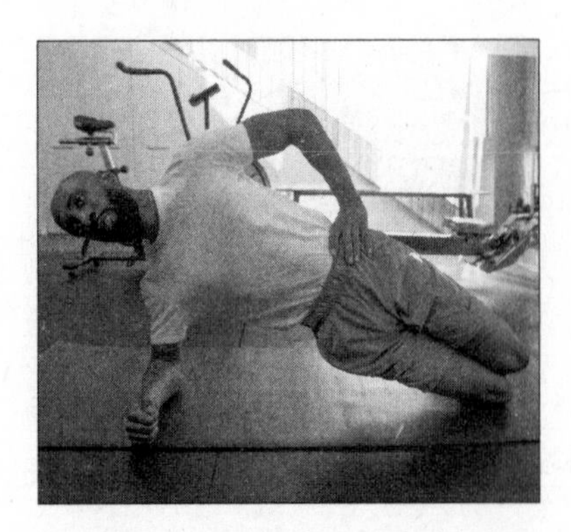

11b. Bent-Knee Side Plank

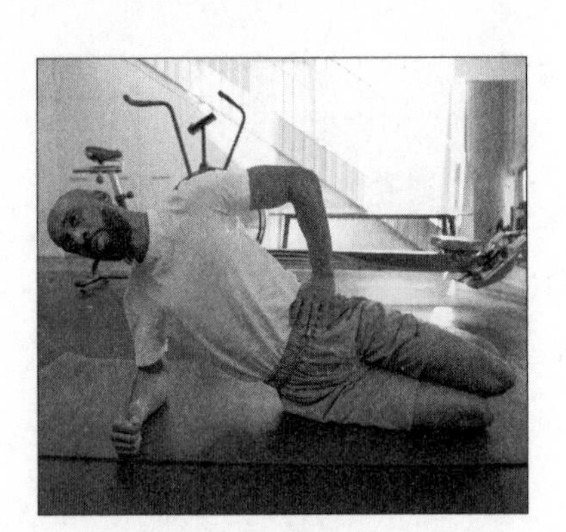

12a. Side Plank with Leg Raise

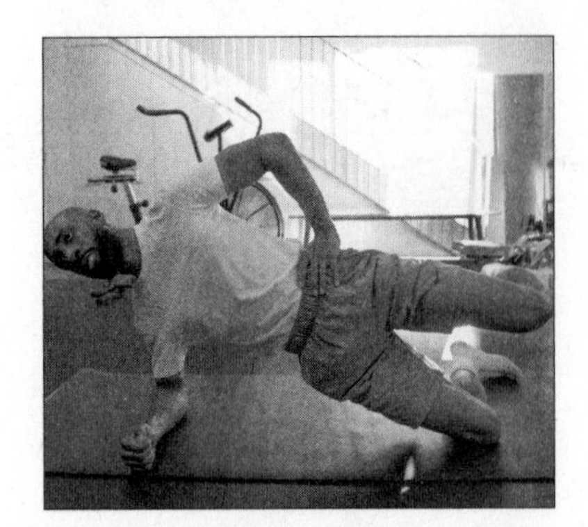

12b. Side Plank with Leg Raise

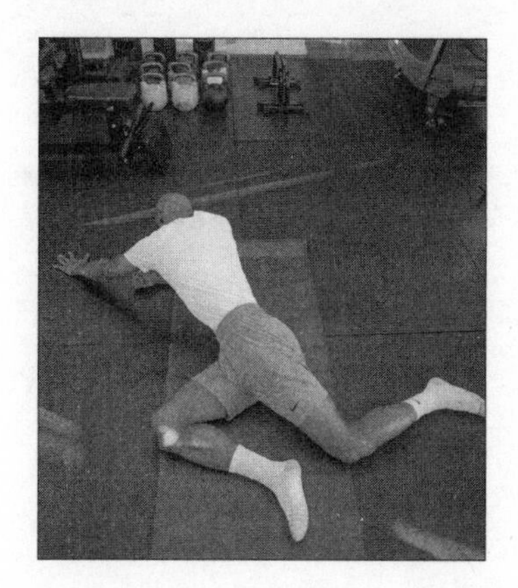

13a. Side Plank March

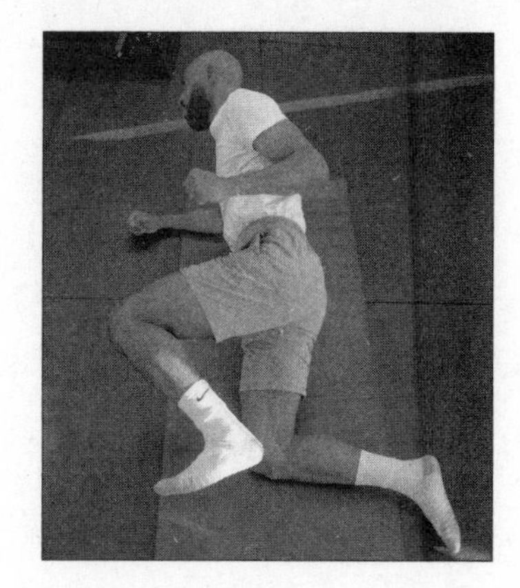

13b. Side Plank March

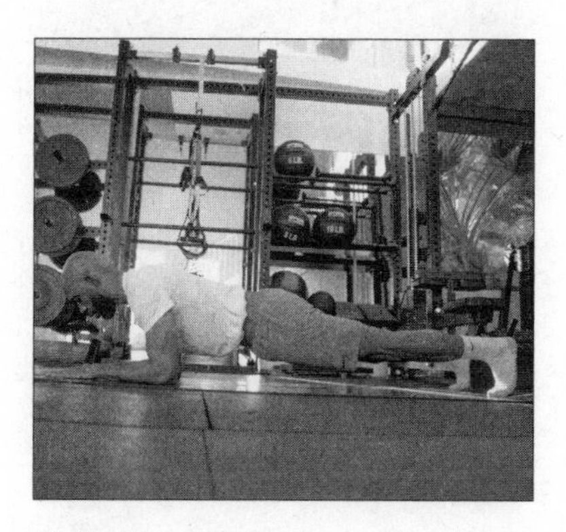

14. Traditional Plank

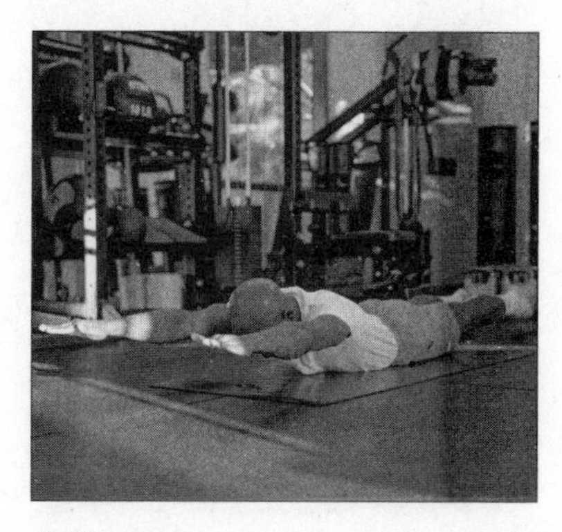

15. Superman

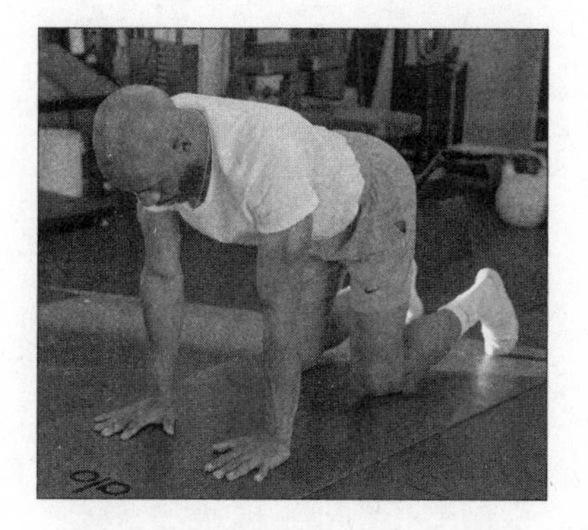

16a. Alternating Arm/Leg Raise

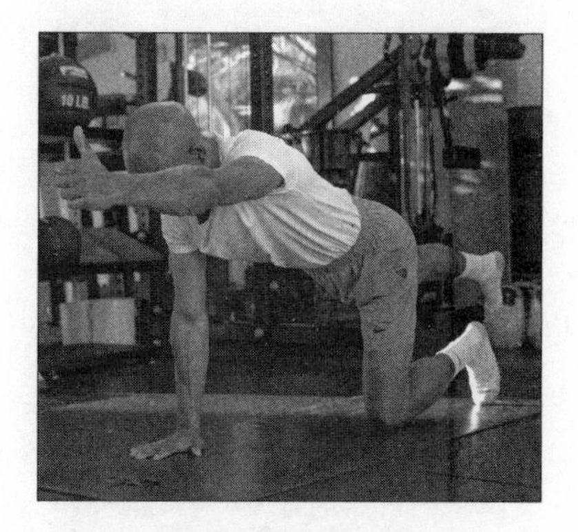

16b. Alternating Arm/Leg Raise

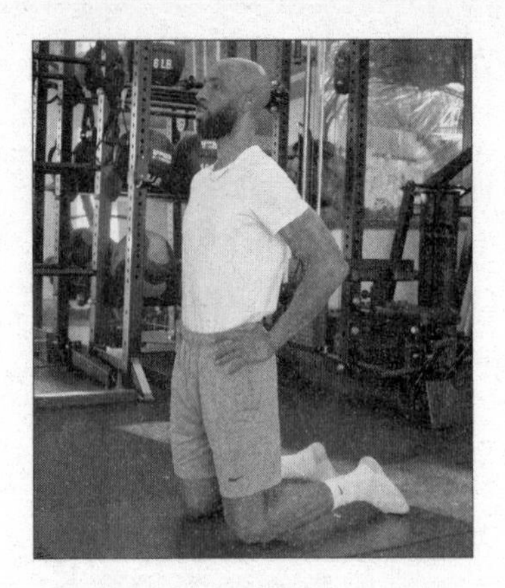

17a. Kneeling Hip Hinge

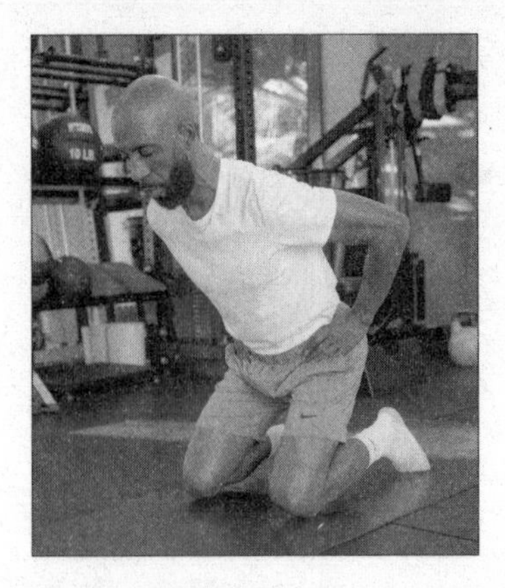

17b. Kneeling Hip Hinge

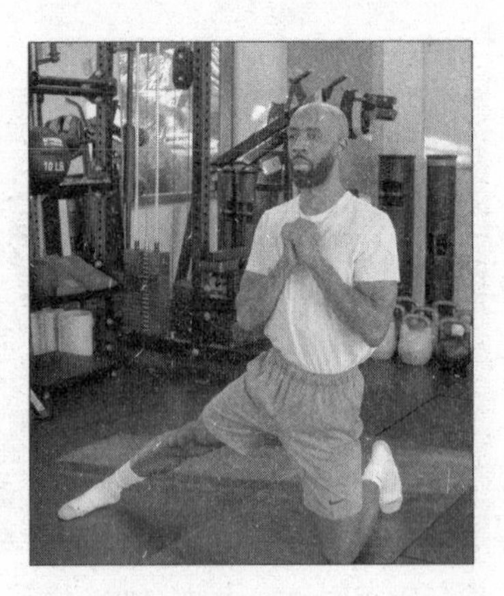

18a. Single-Leg Hip Hinge

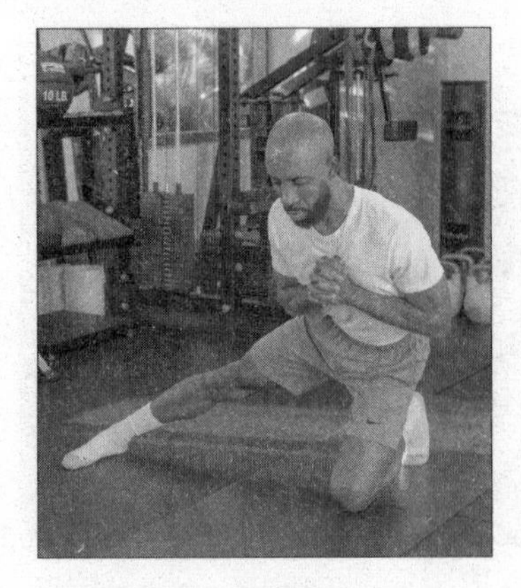

18b. Single-Leg Hip Hinge

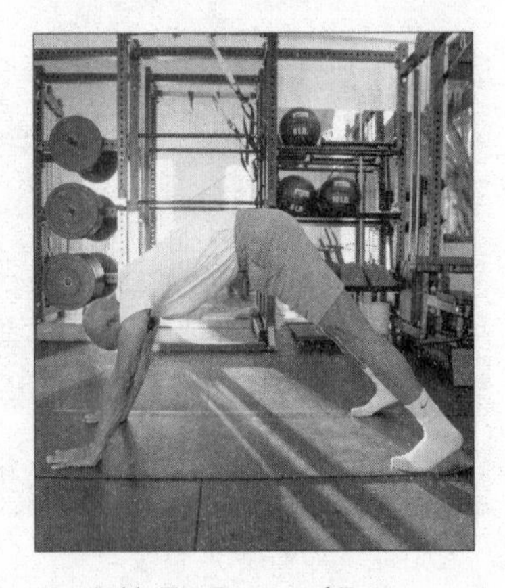

19a. Ankle-Tap Downward Dog

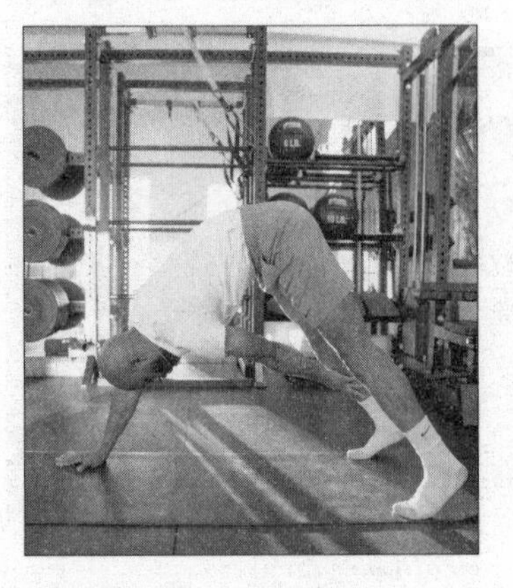

19b. Ankle-Tap Downward Dog

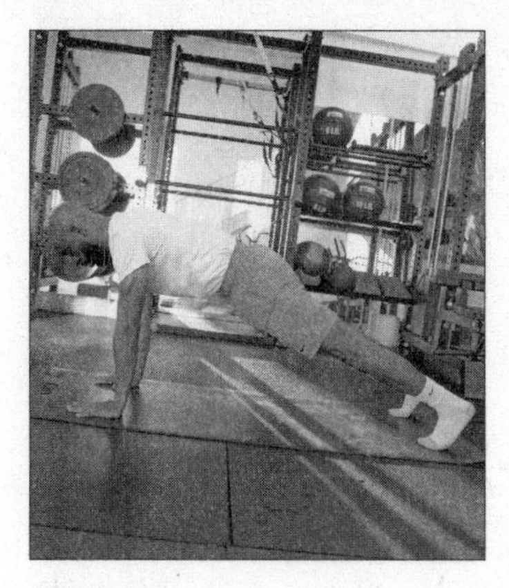

20a. Spider-Man Stretch

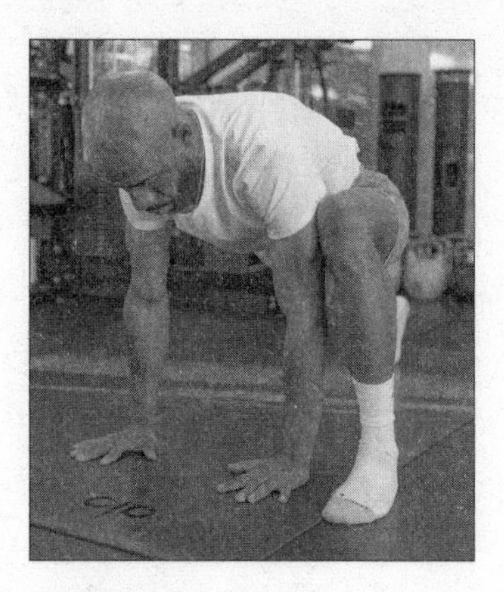

20b. Spider-Man Stretch

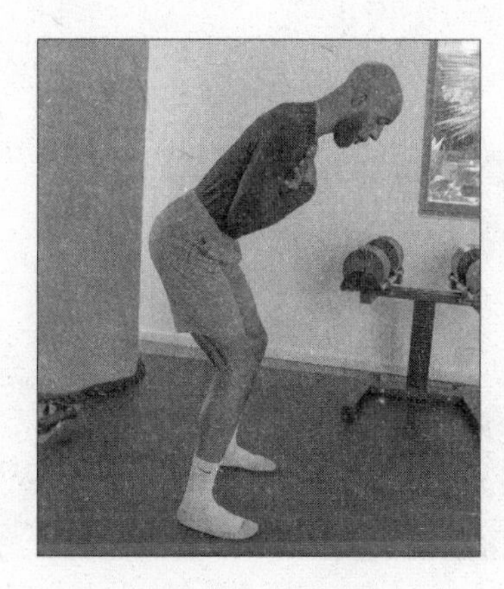

21. Standing Pelvic Tilt

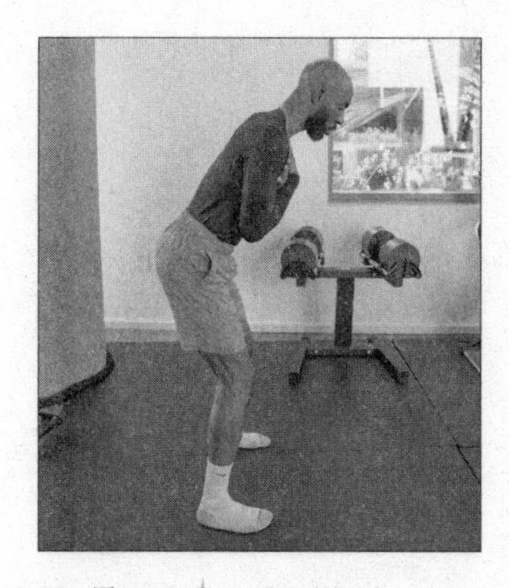

22a. Thoracic Spine Rotation

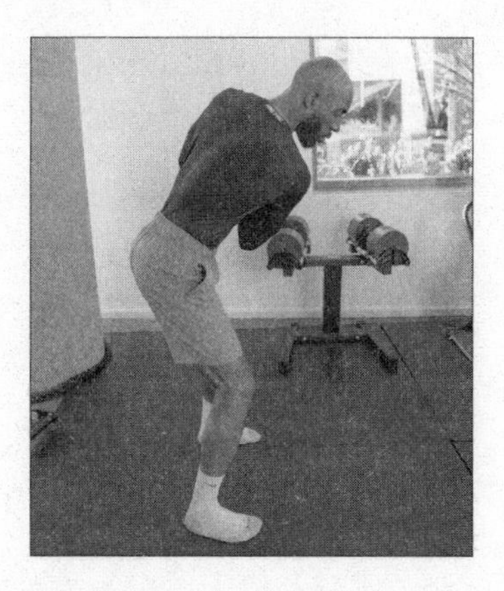

22b. Thoracic Spine Rotation

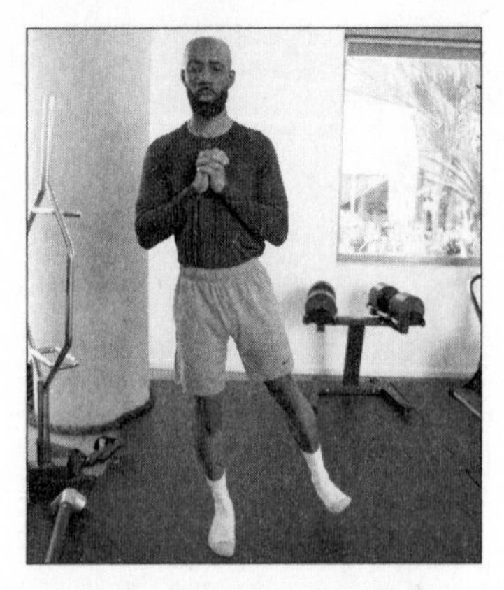

23a. Single-Leg Balance Oscillation

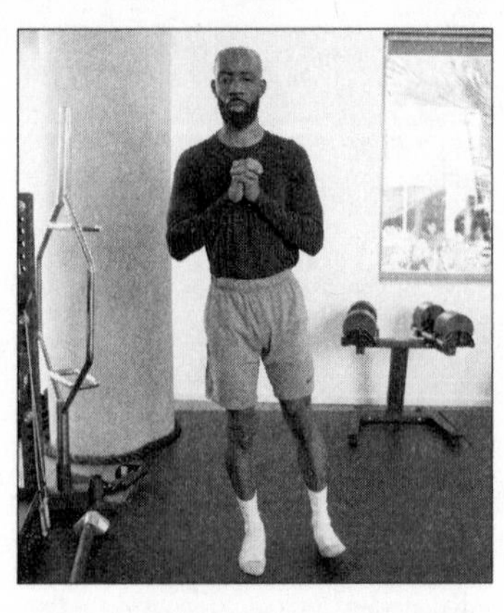

23b. Single-Leg Balance Oscillation

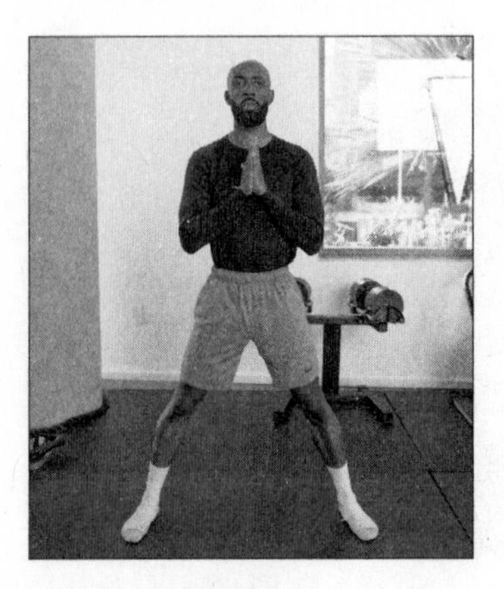

24a. Sumo Lateral Squat

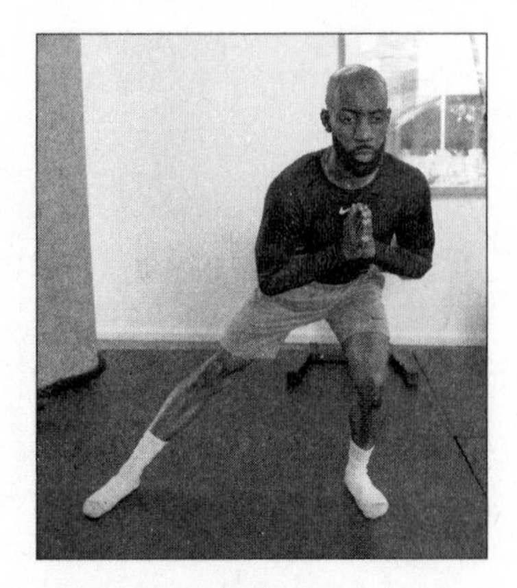

24b. Sumo Lateral Squat

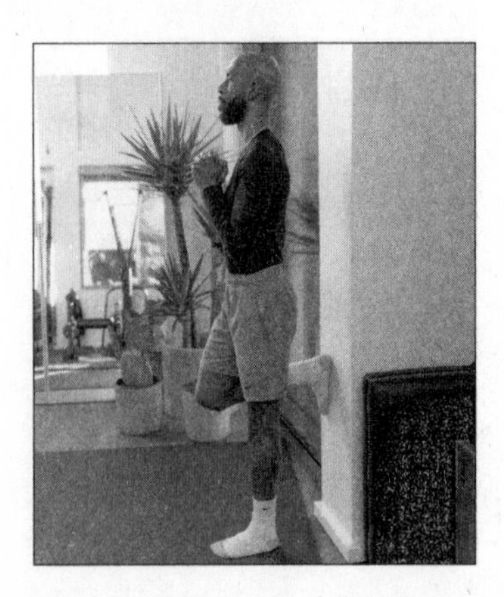

25a. Split-Stance Isometric Wall Squat

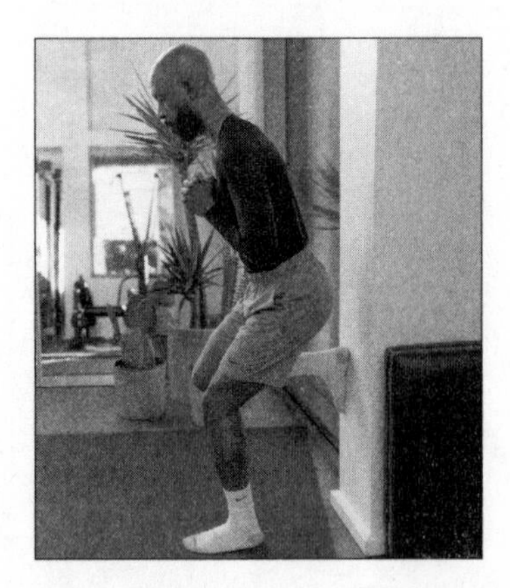

25b. Split-Stance Isometric Wall Squat

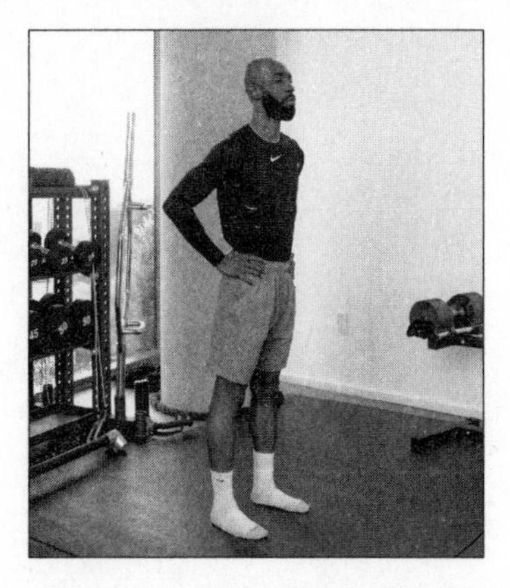

26a. Single-Leg Romanian Deadlift (RDL)

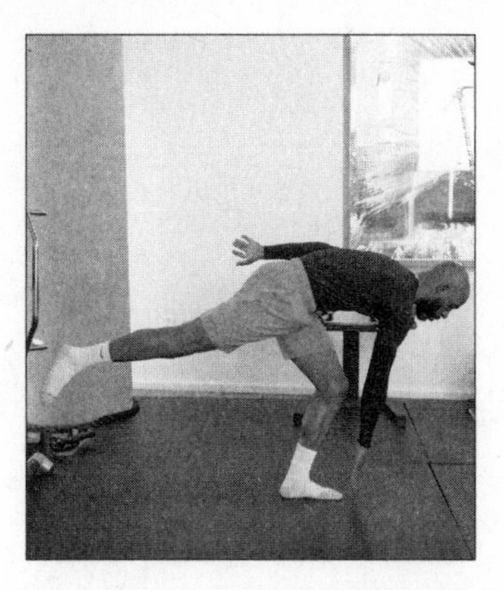

26b. Single-Leg Romanian Deadlift (RDL)

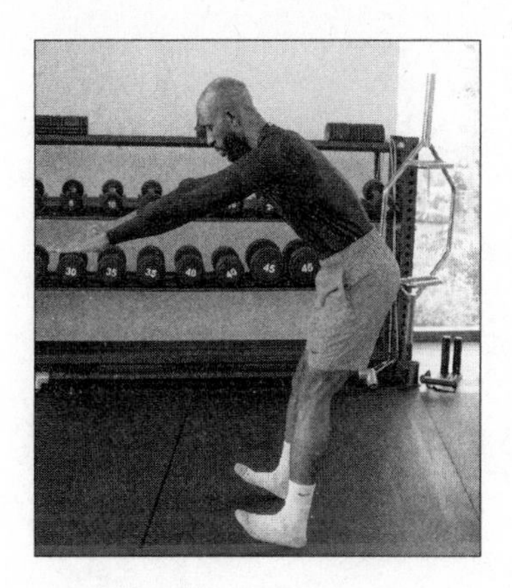

27a. Rocket Ship

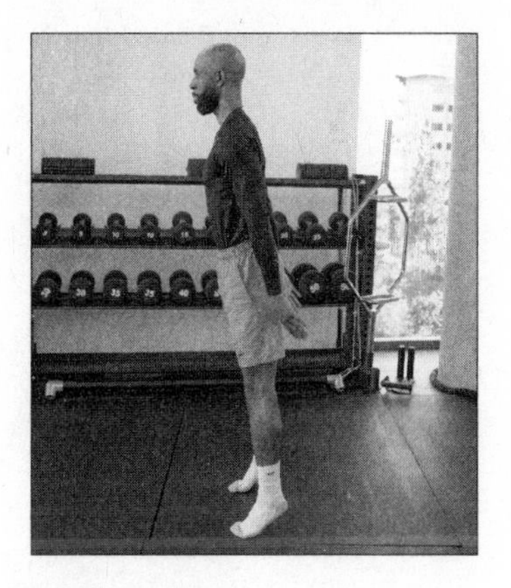

27b. Rocket Ship

For supplementary material from Mike Mancias, please visit:

Acknowledgments

The process of creating a project like this is never done single-handedly. Throughout my life I've been blessed to learn from and be around some great people, and it was with the help of these incredible folks *Game Plan* came to life . . .

- Fara Leff, thank you and the Klutch family for starting all this with the famous "Hey, you should write a book" conversation in your office many moons ago.
- Byrd and my friends at UTA for understanding and supporting me to make this project become a reality.
- Nick and the staff at HarperCollins Publishing for seeing the potential of this project and attacking it!
- Dr. Kevin Marryshow, Darrell Ann, Vinny, and Roy—the team behind the dream that helped put this project together! Thank you.
- Chef Mary Shenouda aka "Paleo Chef"—always appreciate your talks and sessions on all things nutrition! Thank you for sharing your knowledge with me and our audience for *Game Plan*!
- Myatt Murphy, without you there is no *Game Plan*. This project could not have happened without your patience, guidance, and insatiable drive for perfection. You took my thoughts, ideas, and principles on human performance and packaged them in a way that would resonate with the world. You're a pro's pro, brother! Thank you!!

LeBron James:

In 2004, you trusted the kid from Brownsville, Texas, with your health and friendship—I'd say it worked out pretty good for the both of us. It has been an absolute honor and privilege working alongside you for two decades as we redefined sports performance training and longevity together! The greatest to ever do it! You are and will always be the blueprint! Love you and the family always! Thank you!

Myles Garrett:

The NFL's Defensive Player of the Year! Our journey together is fresh—and we are only scratching the surface of the greatness that awaits you. I thank you, Shey, and the Garrett family for your trust and friendship as we navigate through the gridiron together.

Usher:

The definition of timeless longevity. Our journey began in 2021, and that summer we showed the great city of Las Vegas what greatness was all about. And after a record-setting Super Bowl LVIII, NFL halftime entertainment will never be the same! "We killed it!" Always thankful for your trust!

- My family of past and present coaches, athletic trainers, physicians, strength coaches, physical therapists, and equipment managers that taught me the "right way" . . .
    - Jim Lancaster, Keith Jones, and Mark Pfeil—thank you!
    - Stan, Geo, and Cobra—thank you!
- The NBATA & the NBSCA for providing a platform and resource for us to prosper in. Always grateful.
- Tim and MJ, thank you for opening your doors at the original HOOPS the Gym in Chicago for me to witness greatness.

- Friends and family of the Rio Grande Valley and South Texas, home will always be home! I hope my journey can inspire others to go after and achieve even the loftiest of goals—even through adversity.
- My GC brothers, thanks for being my guinea pigs throughout college and beyond! Love y'all.
- Mom, JC, and Luis, your everlasting and unconditional love and support throughout the ups and downs of my journey has meant everything. Love you.
- Heather, Malcolm, and Monica, the three people who sacrifice the most by sharing their husband and daddy with some of the greatest athletes and entertainers in the world—every day! No matter the accolades, you are my greatest achievement! Thank you for your love, understanding, and patience. I know it hasn't been easy. You are my GOATs!

Notes

CHAPTER 4: Follow It Through

1. J. P. Chen, G. C. Chen, X. P. Wang, L. Qin, Y. Bai. Dietary Fiber and Metabolic Syndrome: A Meta-Analysis and Review of Related Mechanisms. *Nutrients,* 2017; 10(1):24. Published 2017 Dec. 26. doi: 10.3390/nu10010024.

2. A. Reynolds, J. Mann, J. Cummings, N. Winter, E. Mete, L. Te Morenga. Carbohydrate Quality and Human Health: A Series of Systematic Reviews and Meta-Analyses. *The Lancet,* 2019 Feb. 2; 393(10170):434–445. Epub 2019 Jan. 10. doi: 10.1016/S0140-6736(18)31809-9.

3. S. McGuire. Scientific Report of the 2015 Dietary Guidelines Advisory Committee. Washington, DC: US Departments of Agriculture and Health and Human Services, 2015. *Advances in Nutrition,* 2016; 7(1):202–204. Published 2016 Jan. 7. doi: 10.3945/an.115.011684.

CHAPTER 6: Rebuild It Better

1. Natalia I. Dmitrieva, Alessandro Gagarin, Delong Liu, Colin O. Wu, Manfred Boehm. Middle-Age High Normal Serum Sodium as a Risk Factor for Accelerated Biological Aging, Chronic Diseases, and Premature Mortality. *eBioMedicine,* 2023; 87:104404. doi: 10.1016/j.ebiom.2022.104404.

2. Yuan-Ting Lo, Yu-Hung Chang, Mark L. Wahlqvist, Han-Bin Huang, Meei-Shyuan Lee. Spending on Vegetable and Fruit Consumption Could Reduce All-Cause Mortality Among Older Adults. *Nutrition Journal,* 2012; 11:113. Published online 2012 Dec. 19. doi: 10.1186/1475-2891-11-113.

CHAPTER 10: Rebuild It Better

1. Farzane Saeidifard, Jose R. Medina-Inojosa, Marta Supervia, Thomas P. Olson, Virend K. Somers, Patricia J. Erwin, Francisco Lopez-Jimenez. Differences of Energy Expenditure While Sitting Versus Standing: A Systematic Review and Meta-Analysis. *European Journal of Preventive Cardiology,* 2018; 25(5):522–538. doi: 10.1177/2047487317752186.

2. L. Yang, C. Cao, E. D. Kantor, et al. Trends in Sedentary Behavior Among the US Population, 2001–2016. *JAMA,* 2019; 321(16):1587–1597. doi: 10.1001/jama.2019.3636.

3. Long H. Nguyen, Po-Hong Liu, Xiaobin Zheng, NaNa Keum, et al. Sedentary Behaviors, TV Viewing Time, and Risk of Young-Onset Colorectal Cancer. *JNCI Cancer Spectrum,* 2018; 2(4). doi: 10.1093/jncics/pky073.

4. University of California–Los Angeles. Sitting Is Bad for Your Brain—Not Just Your Metabolism or Heart: Thinning in Brain Regions Important for Memory Linked to Sedentary Habits. *ScienceDaily,* 2018 Apr. 12. Retrieved May 6, 2019, www.sciencedaily.com/releases/2018/04/180412141014.htm.

5. A. H. Shadyab, C. A. Macera, R. A. Shaffer, S. Jain, et al. Associations of Accelerometer-Measured and Self-Reported Sedentary Time with Leukocyte Telomere Length in Older Women. *American Journal of Epidemiology,* 2017 Feb. 1; 185(3):172–184. doi: 10.1093/aje/kww196.

6. M. L. Larouche, S. L. Mullane, M. J. L. Toledo, M. A. Pereira, J. L. Huberty, B. E. Ainsworth, M. P. Buman. Using Point-of-Choice Prompts to Reduce Sedentary Behavior in Sit-Stand Workstation Users. *Frontiers in Public Health,* 2018 Nov. 21; 6:323. doi: 10.3389/fpubh.2018.00323.

7. T. A. Lakka, D. E. Laaksonen. Physical Activity in Prevention and Treatment of the Metabolic Syndrome. *Applied Physiology, Nutrition, and Metabolism,* 2007 Feb.; 32(1):76–88.

8. Ian Janssen, Valerie Carson, I-Min Lee, Peter T. Katzmarzyk, Steven N. Blair. Years of Life Gained Due to Leisure-Time Physical Activity in the U.S. *American Journal of Preventive Medicine,* 2013. doi: 10.1016/j.amepre.2012.09.056.

9. M. Iwane, M. Arita, S. Tomimoto, O. Satani, M. Matsumoto, K. Miyashita, I. Nishio. Walking 10,000 Steps/Day or More Reduces Blood Pressure and Sympathetic Nerve Activity in Mild Essential Hypertension. *Hypertension Research,* 2000 Nov.; 23(6):573–580.

10. C. H. Yang, D. E. Conroy. Momentary Negative Affect Is Lower During Mindful Movement Than While Sitting: An Experience Sampling Study. *Psychology of Sport and Exercise,* 2018; 37:109–116. doi: 10.1016/j.psychsport.2018.05.003.

CHAPTER 12: **Follow It Through**

1. Luciana Besedovsky, Stoyan Dimitrov, Jan Born, Tanja Lange. Nocturnal Sleep Uniformly Reduces Numbers of Different T-Cell Subsets in the Blood of Healthy Men. *American Journal of Physiology—Regulatory, Integrative and Comparative Physiology,* 2016; 311(4): R637.

2. *Elsevier.* Loss of Sleep, Even for a Single Night, Increases Inflammation in the Body. *ScienceDaily,* 2008 Sept. 4. www.sciencedaily.com/releases/2008/09/080902075211.htm.

3. M. R. Irwin, R. Olmstead, J. E. Carroll. Sleep Disturbance, Sleep Duration, and Inflammation: A Systematic Review and Meta-Analysis of Cohort Studies and Experimental Sleep Deprivation. *Biological Psychiatry,* 2016 July 1; 80(1):40–52. doi: 10.1016/j.biopsych.2015.05.014.

4. Radiological Society of North America. Short-Term Sleep Deprivation Affects Heart Function. *ScienceDaily,* 2016 Dec. 2.

5. Graham H. Diering, Raja S. Nirujogi, Richard H. Roth, Paul F. Worley, Akhilesh Pandey, Richard L. Huganir. Homer1a Drives Homeostatic Scaling-Down of Excitatory Synapses During Sleep, *Science,* 2017 Feb. 2; 355(6324):511–515..

6. H. K. Al Khatib, S. V. Harding, J. Darzi, G. K. Pot. The Effects of Partial Sleep Deprivation on Energy Balance: A Systematic Review and Meta-Analysis. *European Journal of Clinical Nutrition,* 2016 Nov. 2.

7. Aric A. Prather, Cindy W. Leung, Nancy E. Adler, Lorrene Ritchie, Barbara Laraia, Elissa S. Epel. Short and Sweet: Associations Between Self-Reported Sleep Duration and Sugar-Sweetened Beverage Consumption Among Adults in the United States. *Sleep Health,* 2016.

8. Jonas Lötscher, Adrià-Arnau Martí i Líndez, Nicole Kirchhammer, Elisabetta Cribioli, et al. Magnesium Sensing via LFA-1 Regulates CD8 T Cell Effector Function. *Cell,* 2022. doi: 10.1016/j.cell.2021.12.039.

9. L. A. Te Morenga, A. J. Howatson, R. M. Jones, J. Mann. Dietary Sugars and Cardiometabolic Risk: Systematic Review and Meta-Analyses of Randomized Controlled Trials of the Effects on Blood Pressure and Lipids. *American Journal of Clinical Nutrition*, 2014; 100(1):65. doi: 10.3945/ajcn.113.081521.

10. G. Howatson, M. P. McHugh, J. A. Hill, et al. Influence of Tart Cherry Juice on Indices of Recovery Following Marathon Running. *Scandinavian Journal of Medicine and Science in Sports*, 2009. doi: 10.1111/j.1600-0838.2009.01005.x.

11. Ivy C. Mason, Daniela Grimaldi, Kathryn J. Reid, et al. Light Exposure During Sleep Impairs Cardiometabolic Function. *Proceedings of the National Academy of Sciences*, 2022; 119(12). doi: 10.1073/pnas.2113290119.

12. Nina C. Franklin, Mohamed M. Ali, Austin T. Robinson, Edita Norkeviciute, Shane A. Phillips. Massage Therapy Restores Peripheral Vascular Function following Exertion. *Archives of Physical Medicine and Rehabilitation*, 2014. doi: 10.1016/j.apmr.2014.02.007.

13. J. D. Crane, D. I. Ogborn, C. Cupido, S. Melov, et al. Massage Therapy Attenuates Inflammatory Signaling After Exercise-Induced Muscle Damage. *Science Translational Medicine*, 2012; 4(119):119ra13. doi: 10.1126/scitranslmed.3002882.

14. Cynthia Marske, Samantha Shah, Aaron Chavira, Caleb Hedberg, et al. Mindfulness-Based Stress Reduction in the Management of Chronic Pain and Its Comorbid Depression. *The Journal of the American Osteopathic Association*, 2020; 120(9):575. doi: 10.7556/jaoa.2020.096.

15. Kimberley Luu, Peter A. Hall. Examining the Acute Effects of Hatha Yoga and Mindfulness Meditation on Executive Function and Mood. *Mindfulness*, 2016; 8(4):873. doi: 10.1007/s12671-016-0661-2.

16. A. C. Hafenbrack, Z. Kinias, S. G. Barsade. Debiasing the Mind Through Meditation: Mindfulness and the Sunk-Cost Bias. *Psychological Science*, 2013; 25(2):369. doi: 10.1177/0956797613503853.

17. S. Pooley, O. Spendiff, M. Allen, H. J. Moir. Comparative Efficacy of Active Recovery and Cold Water Immersion as Post-Match Recovery Interventions in Elite Youth Soccer. *Journal of Sports Sciences*, 2020 June; 38(11–12):1423–1431. Epub 2019 Aug. 28. doi: 10.1080/02640414.2019.1660448.

18. Micah Allen, Somogy Varga, Detlef H. Heck. Respiratory Rhythms of the Predictive Mind. *Psychological Review*, 2022. doi: 10.1037/rev0000391.

19. Michael Christopher Melnychuk, Paul M. Dockree, Redmond G. O'Connell, Peter R. Murphy, Joshua H. Balsters, Ian H. Robertson. Coupling of Respiration and Attention via the Locus Coeruleus: Effects of Meditation and Pranayama. *Psychophysiology*, 2018; e13091. doi: 10.1111/psyp.13091.

CHAPTER 14: Rebuild It Better

1. W. L. Haskell, I. M. Lee, R. R. Pate, et al. Physical Activity and Public Health: Updated Recommendation for Adults from the American College of Sports Medicine and the American Heart Association. *Medicine & Science in Sports & Exercise*, 2007 Aug.; 39(8):1423–1434.

2. T. M. Eijsvogels, P. D. Thompson. Exercise Is Medicine: At Any Dose? *JAMA*, 2015 Nov. 10; 314(18):1915–1916. doi: 10.1001/jama.2015.10858.

3. Brice Faraut, Samir Nakib, Catherine Drogou, Maxime Elbaz, et al. Napping Reverses the Salivary Interleukin-6 and Urinary Norepinephrine Changes Induced by Sleep Restriction. *The Journal of Clinical Endocrinology & Metabolism*, 2015; 100(3):E416–426. doi: 10.1210/jc.2014-2566.

4. Sara Studte, Emma Bridger, Axel Mecklinger. Nap Sleep Preserves Associative but Not Item Memory Performance. *Neurobiology of Learning and Memory*, 2015; 120: 84. doi: 10.1016/j.nlm.2015.02.012.

5. Valentina Paz, Hassan S. Dashti, Victoria Garfield. Is There an Association Between Daytime Napping, Cognitive Function, and Brain Volume? A Mendelian

Randomization Study in the UK Biobank. *Sleep Health*, 2023. doi: 10.1016/j.sleh.2023.05.002.

6. Bodil Ekholm, Stefan Spulber, Mats Adler. A Randomized Controlled Study of Weighted Chain Blankets for Insomnia in Psychiatric Disorders. *Journal of Clinical Sleep Medicine*, 2020; 16(9):1567.doi: 10.5664/jcsm.8636.